Project ReBuild

C.R. Escobar, M.Msc.

This publication is designed to provide information regarding the subject matter covered. However, laws and practices often vary from state to state and are subject to change. Because each factual situation is different, specific advice should be tailored to the particular circumstances. For this reason, the reader is advised to consult with his or her own advisor or medical provider regarding their specific situation.

The author has taken reasonable precautions in the preparation of this book and believe the facts in the book are accurate as of the date it was written. However, the author assumes no responsibility for any errors or omissions. The author specifically disclaims any liability resulting from the use or application of the information contained in this book, and the information is not intended to serve as legal, financial, medical or other professional advice related to individual situations.

Published by Christine R Escobar

FIRST EDITION

Cover Design by Susan Blanchard
Pictures by Unsplash, Pexels, and Pixabay

ISBN: 9798553239626

Mydynamiclife.org

Disclaimer

All content found in Project Rebuild, including: text, images, audio, or other formats were created for informational purposes only. The content is not intended to be a substitute for professional medical advice, diagnosis, or treatment. Always seek the advice of your physician or other qualified health provider with any questions you may have regarding a medical condition. Never disregard professional medical advice or delay in seeking it because of something you have read in any of Project Rebuild's content (books, Facebook page, website, YouTube, etc.)

If you think you may have a medical emergency, call your doctor, go to the emergency department, or call 911 immediately. Project Rebuild does not recommend or endorse any specific tests, physicians, products, procedures, opinions, or other information that may be mentioned. Reliance on any information provided by Project Rebuild is solely at your own risk.

Links to additional content not created by Project Rebuild are taken at your own risk. Project Rebuild is not responsible for the claims of external websites and educational companies or providers.

Table of Contents

We have beat breast cancer.

Now what?

We endured the emotional roller coaster ride; tears, fears, anger, laughter and love.

Our bodies have gone through hell. Chemo. Exhaustion. Nausea. Hair loss. Radiation. Mastectomy.

Some of us were thrown into a chemo-induced menopause. Talk about going from 100 mph to a complete stop in an instant!

So, now what?

Most of us are now on a hormone blocker or aromatase inhibitors. Some doctors say five years. Other doctors say ten years. Even the dose of the medication is different.

What does this mean for us? For you? For me?

Hello… It's me.

It was November 10, 2017, the day before Veteran's Day. I had just experienced my first mammogram and found myself sitting in a hospital gown in a cold, sterile room full of machines. I was told to wait while she spoke with the doctor. As I sat there, I began to think, "This is taking longer than I expected. She's taking too long. The technician has been gone too long." Dread came over me, and I silently braced myself for the actual diagnosis.

So many of us have a story like this to tell. Most of us will *never* forget the date, time and place. At some point, I felt like I was moving through water; like walking through a swimming pool. We all have our cancer stories, and each journey is similar but unique to you. Now that the horrors of chemotherapy and surgery have ended, we have been placed on a different kind of drug; a hormone blocker. The side effects are astounding and can be debilitating.

With extreme bone pain, and unlimitless fatigue, I started researching this stuff. Are there other women going through this too? What if I *don't* take this stuff? What is the probability of my cancer coming back if I stop taking this medicine? Am I the only one gaining so much weight? Is there a natural alternative? I really didn't want to feel the need for a walker while still in my 40's. The questions flooded my fuzzy, chemo brain as I desperately searched for answers.

I eventually found a few chat rooms filled with women from around the world with the same questions and experiences. Many questions went unanswered. Some questions dated back to 2010, and are still unanswered. No one had answers, but every woman supported, and encouraged one another. I began looking for books, websites, scientific reports, clinical trials, anything… I felt desperate. Well, I didn't find everything in one spot, but I did find lots of answers scattered across the internet. So, I've put all those answers together in one place for all of us.

Let me make something clear though… I am not a doctor. I am not a nurse. I am not a scientist. I am a woman that went through breast cancer that did a lot of research. I am not saying that any of this will work for you. I am not saying any of this information is a miracle cure. I'm not telling you to stop taking your medication, to reduce your medication or change your medication. It's still very important to discuss all your questions about your treatment with your provider and come up with a plan that is best suited for you and your body. All information has a link to the actual website, report, etc. for your further review and research at the end under "Resources". This is my disclosure *again*, so don't come after me if something goes wrong.

Christine R Escobar

Part 1: the Project

Chemo-Induced Menopause or Medical Menopause

I never really knew this existed until it happened to me. Isn't that how it usually works anyway? The light bulb goes off and the infamous, "ohhh… I get it now!" is uttered in complete wonder. I look back at the side effects I had during my treatments. I'm realizing now that those side effects were probably symptoms of menopause.

MD Anderson in Houston, TX explains it best: "Chemotherapy fights cancer by attacking any rapidly growing cells. Women receiving chemotherapy – regardless of the type of cancer they've been diagnosed with – are at risk of the drugs attacking the ovaries. 'Chemotherapy basically puts the ovaries to sleep,' Lim says. The ovaries stop processing the eggs, the woman stops having a period and she goes into temporary menopause.

In most cases, menstruation returns naturally eight months to two years after chemotherapy stops. However, research shows that women who experience temporary menopause during treatment tend to go into complete menopause earlier than others. 'But it really depends on the patient,' Lim adds.

However, if a woman is already nearing menopause, chemotherapy may put her into complete menopause and her period may never return. *Menopausal symptoms can seem more exaggerated in breast cancer patients* (emphasis mine). When it occurs naturally, menopause takes a few years from the time your period gets interrupted to the time it completely stops. But cancer treatment can speed up the process so that it takes only a few months.

To help lower hormone levels after cancer treatment, many women undergo hormone therapy. Also known as endocrine therapy, it works by either blocking the hormones or by preventing the body from making them. Examples of hormone therapies include tamoxifen, raloxifene, ovarian suppression injections and aromatase inhibitors." (Menopause – MD Anderson)

Estrogen

The word "Estrogen" has become such a "bad" word, it seems, especially in the breast cancer world. It makes me sad. Estrogen is what makes us women. So, why does it have to be so taboo? If we take all our estrogen away, what are the long term effects? Are there any positive effects of our beloved hormone? Dr. Jeffrey D. Blaustein explains what estrogen really is and how it works.

"There is actually no hormone called 'estrogen'. Estrogens are a class of hormones. There are three different forms of estrogens in the body: estradiol, estriol and estrone. Although they are all pretty similar in function, they vary in potency. Estrogens found in plants, like soy, are also sometimes simply called "estrogen," although their effects may differ from those of the estrogens produced in the body.

Estradiol is the dominant estrogen circulating prior to menopause. It is produced mainly in the ovaries. In most cases, this is the most potent form of estrogen. During pregnancy, the dominant form is estriol, produced by the placenta. And during menopause, when the levels of estradiol decrease, the dominant estrogen is estrone, produced in fat tissue." (Estrogen – the Conversation)

We all know that estrogens are responsible for puberty, the reproductive system, and our sexuality. But, did you know that estrogen regulates our temperature? That's where the hot flashes come in. It also influences our brain; how we think, our memory, and how we express ourselves through language. It's also considered an antidepressant, helps us sleep, influences our sexual desire, maintains bone density, and may even decrease the possibility of Alzheimer's disease. Isn't that amazing?

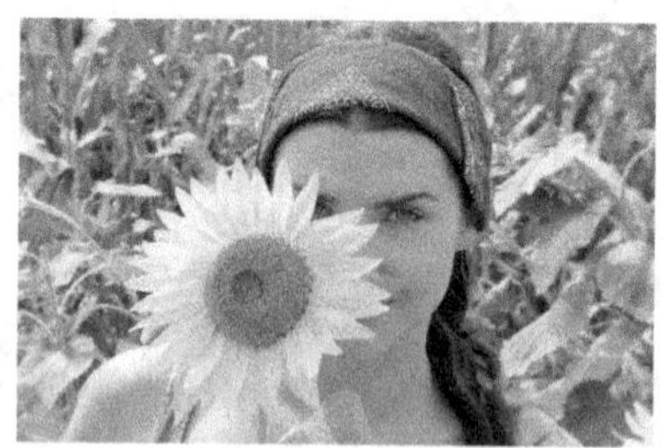

Phytoestrogens

What are phytoestrogens? Are they safe for breast cancer patients? Are they a risk? Or are they beneficial?

"A 2009 study found that consuming soy foods decreased the risk of death and recurrence in women with breast cancer. Soy foods are rich in phytoestrogens.
Another study in 2015, found that phytoestrogens inhibited the growth of breast cancer cells. A further study suggested the role of phytoestrogens in breast cancer survival is complex and depends on what stage of menopause a woman is in.
Phytoestrogens are not appropriate for all types of cancer. Anyone considering taking phytoestrogens should discuss it with their doctor first." (Phytoestrogens – Medical News Today)

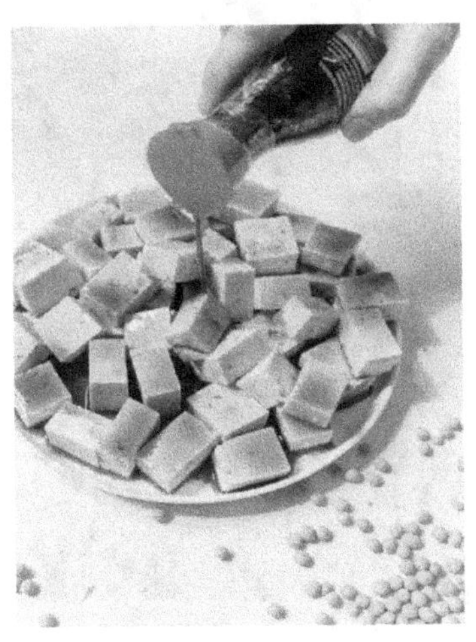

Black Cohosh:

Some women with breast cancer use this herb to help control menopausal symptoms caused by their treatment, but research is inconsistent on the scientific evidence. It's advised that "women who have breast cancer, who have had breast cancer in the past or are at high-risk for breast cancer, should avoid Black Cohosh". (Black Cohosh – Komen)

On the other hand, this clinical trial shows that "current evidence does not support an association between black cohosh and increased risk of breast cancer." (Black Cohosh – PubMed NCBI)

I, personally, don't take it. I'd rather be safe than sorry.

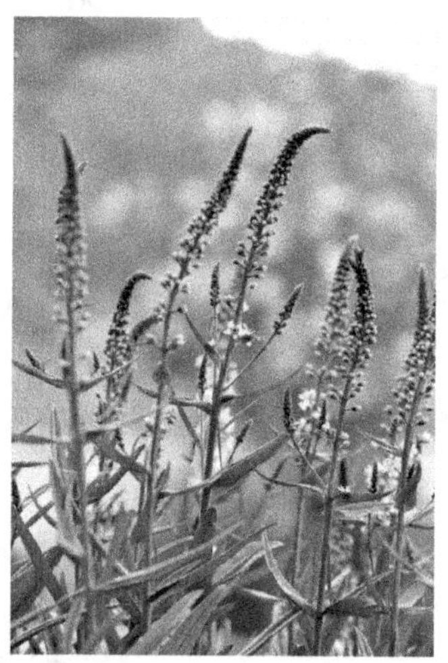

Red Clover:

"Researchers have begun to study the role of isoflavones from red clover in cancer prevention and treatment. Preliminary evidence suggests these isoflavones may stop cancer cells from growing or kill cancer cells in test tubes. However, because of the herb's estrogen-like effects, it might also contribute to the growth of some cancers, just as estrogen does. Until further research is done, doctors cannot recommend red clover to prevent cancer. Women with a history of breast cancer should not take red clover." (Red Clover – Penn State Hershey) (Red Clover – MSKCC)

I don't take this herb either.

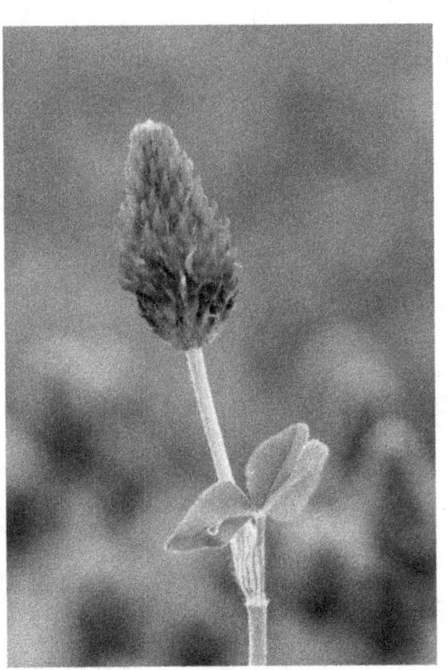

Soy Isoflavones:

Can I eat soy products or not? One study says it's good for cancer patients. The next study says it actually causes the very cancer we're trying to avoid. So which is it?

This is what the American Cancer Society has to say about it. "In human studies, the estrogen effects of soy seem to either have no effect at all, or to reduce breast cancer risk. This may be because the isoflavones can actually block the more potent natural estrogens in the blood. So far, the evidence does not point to any dangers from eating soy in people, and the health benefits appear to outweigh any potential risk. There is growing evidence that eating traditional soy foods (tofu, edamame, miso and soy milk) may lower the risk of breast cancer." (Soy – cancer.org)

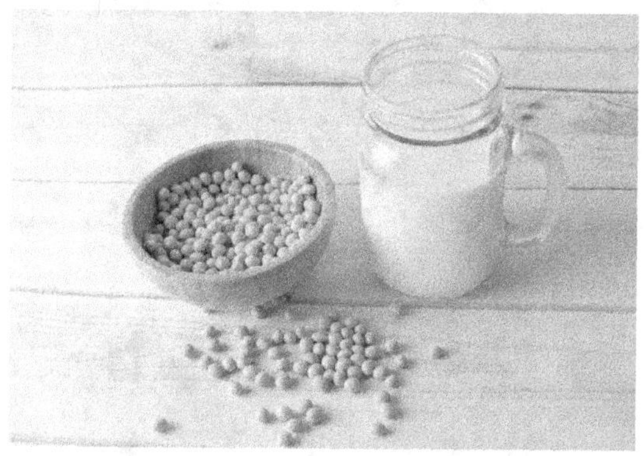

Dong Quai:

"If you have a hormone-sensitive cancer, this herb has estrogenic effects and can further stimulate the growth of cancer cells. If you are undergoing radiation therapy, dong quai can cause photo dermatitis, and therefore might worsen the effects of radiation therapy on the skin." (Dong Quai – MSKCC)

Ginseng:

"American ginseng has not been shown to treat or prevent cancer. Breast cancer patients should use this herb with caution because it can stimulate the growth of breast cancer cells." (Ginseng – MSKCC)

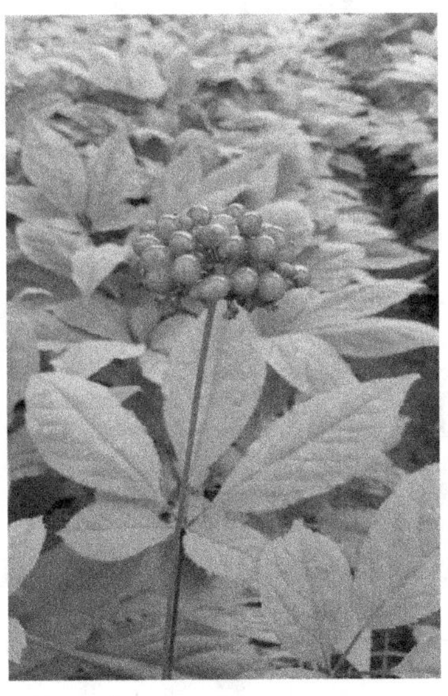

Anti-Hormone Therapy

I say "Anti-Hormone Therapy" because it's our hormones that has caused this big mess in the first place! And Hormone *Replacement* Therapy (HRT) is clearly not allowed!
Anti-hormone therapy is best for hormone positive breast cancer patients and the treatment depends on whether you're pre-menopausal or post-menopausal. I was perimenopausal when I started my chemo treatments. Chemotherapy pushed me into menopause. After an official one year of no menstruation, I was considered officially post-menopausal. With that, I've been placed on an aromatase inhibitor (Letrozole/Femara) rather than Tamoxifen. My doctor had initially wanted to put me on Tamoxifen. Due to my history of blood clots, I researched the medication and discovered it can cause stroke or pulmonary embolism and so on. Just remember, there's nothing wrong with questioning your doctor about alternate medications or procedures. You're paying them for a service and a healthy payment at that!

I'm sure you have already researched and read through all the side effects that *your* medication warrants. I know you've discussed this in great detail with your doctor. I did the same. But, I always have this nagging feeling that the doctor doesn't always tell me everything. Now, I could get into "big pharma" and the greed for money, etc. but the bottom line is that I just really want to know what my body is being subjected to. If I know most of the side effects, then I can determine if it's really the medication or if it's possibly something else. My initial oncologist reduced the dosage, so my quality of life would be better. My current doctor wants me to take the full dose. I tried and I felt like I needed a walker. I'm not a doctor, but the way I see it… as long as I have it in my system, I should be good. So, I cut all my pills in a half.

*I'm not saying this is what *you* should do. I'm saying this is what works for *me*.*

My "go-to" site for all medications is https://www.drugs.com/.
They give you the entire breakdown of whatever your doctor wants
to give; the warning, reviews, images, side effects, the science, and so
on. There's even a breakdown of the side effects based on the
immediate need for medical attention and how common, less
common or rare it is. The information for each medication listed
here is directly from drugs.com. I've included a direct link for
further research.

Other websites for medication research include
https://www.rxlist.com and https://www.pdr.net/

Selective Estrogen Receptor Modulators (SERM)

"Selective estrogen receptor modulators, called SERMs for short, block the effects of estrogen in the breast tissue. SERMs work by sitting in the estrogen receptors in breast cells. If a SERM is in the estrogen receptor, there is no room for estrogen and it can't attach to the cell. If estrogen isn't attached to a breast cell, the cell doesn't receive estrogen's signals to grow and multiply."
"Cells in other tissues in the body, such as bones and the uterus, also have estrogen receptors. But each estrogen receptor has a slightly different structure, depending on the kind of cell it is in. So breast cell estrogen receptors are different from bone cell estrogen receptors and both of those estrogen receptors are different from uterine estrogen receptors. As their name says, SERMs are "selective" — this means that a SERM that blocks estrogen's action in breast cells can activate estrogen's action in other cells, such as bone, liver, and uterine cells." (Breast cancer - serms)
So, for women that are still in their child-bearing years, this is the best plan of action.

Tamoxifen (Soltamox)

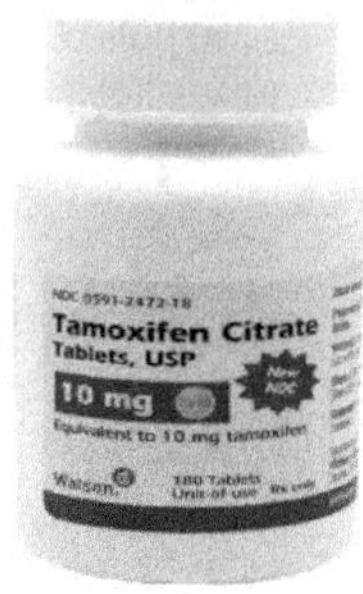

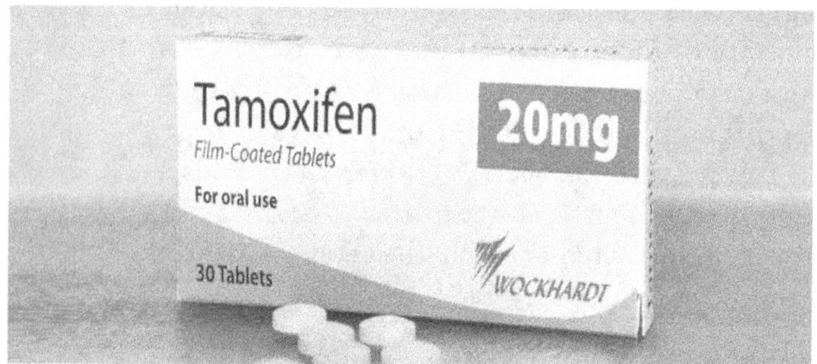

Toremifene (Fareston)

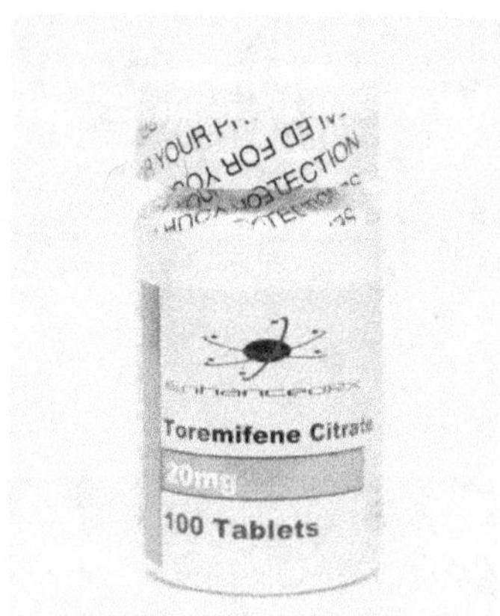

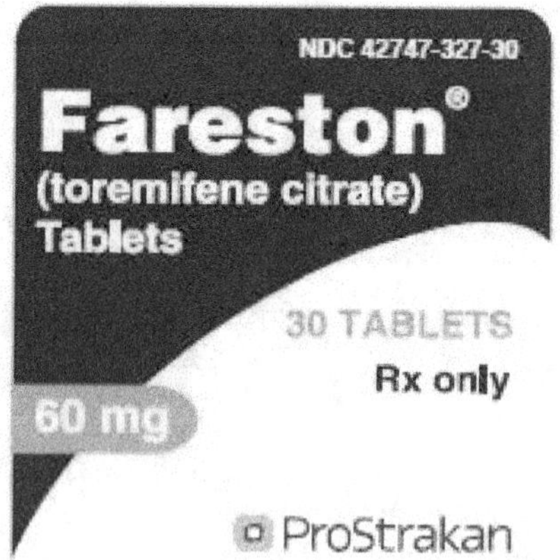

Fulvestrant (Faslodex)

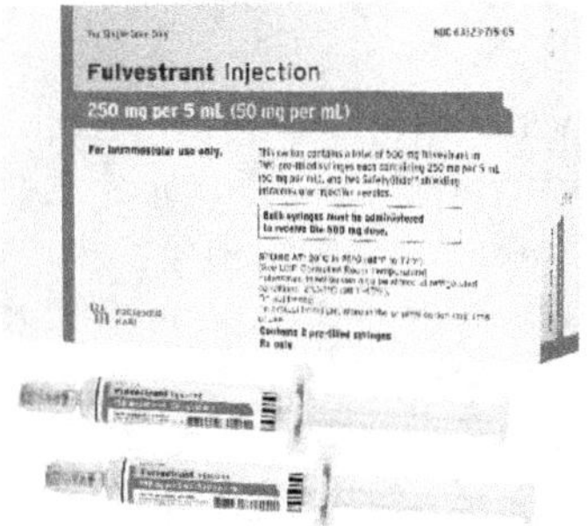

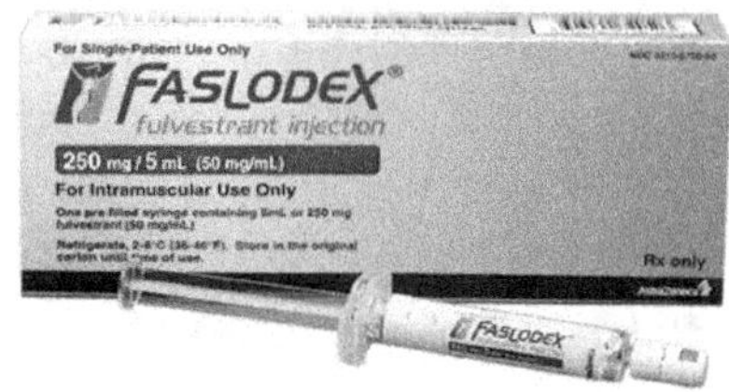

Aromatase Inhibitors (AI)

"Aromatase inhibitors stop the production of estrogen in postmenopausal women. Aromatase inhibitors work by blocking the enzyme aromatase, which turns the hormone androgen into small amounts of estrogen in the body. This means that less estrogen is available to stimulate the growth of hormone-receptor-positive breast cancer cells. Aromatase inhibitors can't stop the ovaries from making estrogen, so aromatase inhibitors are mainly used to treat postmenopausal women." (breast cancer – ai)

For women that are already post-menopausal, this is our best plan of action. This was one of my biggest questions, and my doctor's didn't give me an answer… If I'm in menopause that means my ovaries are no longer active or producing any estrogen; so why am I taking a hormone blocker? The answer: "Although the ovaries no longer make large amounts of estrogen, male hormones (androgens) do circulate in the blood and can be changed into estrogen. An enzyme called aromatase carries out this change."
(URMC Rochester)

In trying to find justification in *not* taking this medication, I found the answer explaining why I *should* take it.

Letrozole (Femara)

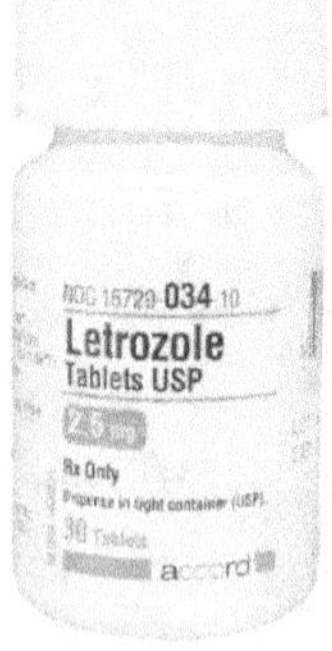

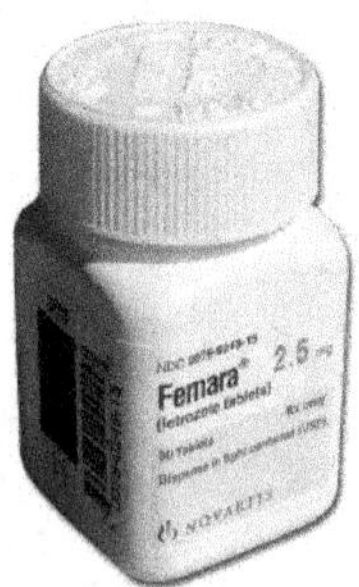

Exemestane (Aromasin)

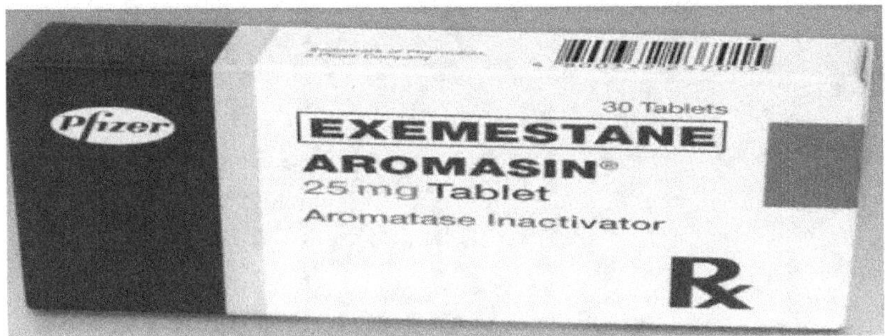

Anastrozole (Arimidex)

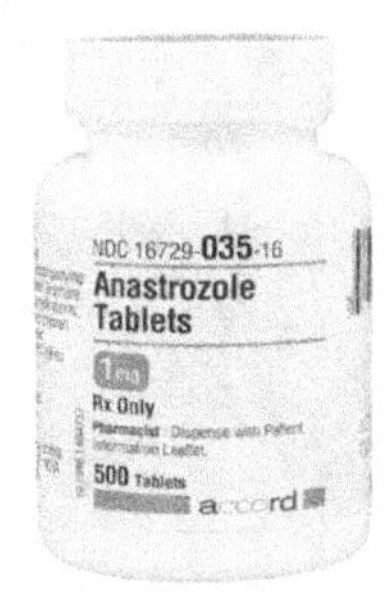

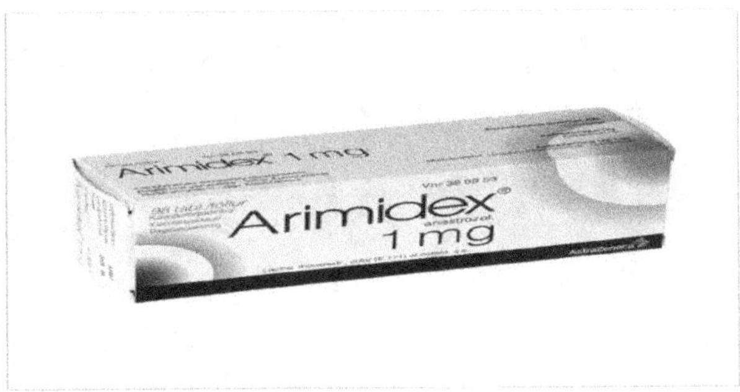

Part 2: Managing Side-Effects

Osteopenia vs. Osteoporosis

Within the last three months, I've moved from one state to another and reestablished new doctors and hospitals despite the craziness of 2020. My new oncologist requested a bone density scan for osteoporosis since it runs in my family. My aromatase inhibitor (Letrozole) can cause it as well. I was surprised my original doctor didn't request one… or maybe she did, but my chemo brain didn't remember! Anyway, my results came back, and I now have Osteopenia. Great. What does that mean?

Let's start with the bone density scan, also known as a DXA or DEXA scan (dual-energy X-ray absorptiometry). The scan measures the bone density in the hip and the spine; which, can predict possible future breaks or fractures in other bones. The test only took about 10-15 minutes. I sat in the waiting room longer than the actual procedure took.

The test results are reported using T-scores. This shows how much your bone density is compared to a healthy 30-year old. The score is based on negative numbers; the closer to 0, the better off you are. See the chart:

Guide to Understanding T-Scores

GUIDE TO UNDERSTANDING T-SCORES

Category	T-scores Range	Examples
Normal Bone Density	-1 and above	+0.5
		0
		-1.0
Low Bone Density (Osteopenia)	Between -1 and -2.5	-1.1
		-1.5
		-2.4
Osteoporosis	-2.5 and below	-2.5
		-3.0
		-4.0

(nof.org – bone-density test)

My score was -1.9 and I'm 49 years old. So now, I question the anti-hormone therapy. Is it worth the risk, taking anti-hormone medicine, to *prevent* a recurrence of breast cancer, despite a double mastectomy? Or do I risk a recurrence of cancer and *not* take anti-hormone therapy in order to prevent osteoporosis and a wheelchair? <heavy sigh>   This is what I found:

When to Consider Treatment

The results of a bone density test help your healthcare provider make recommendations about what you can do to reduce your chance of breaking a bone. When making a decision about treatment with an osteoporosis medicine, your healthcare provider will also consider your risk factors for osteoporosis, your likelihood of breaking a bone in the future, your medical history and your current health.

Below are treatment guidelines for postmenopausal women and men age 50 or older:
Most people with T-scores of -1.0 and above (normal bone density) do not need to take an osteoporosis medicine.
Some people with T-scores between -1.0 and -2.5 (low bone density or osteopenia) should consider taking an osteoporosis medicine when they have certain risk factors.
All people with T-scores of -2.5 and below (osteoporosis) should consider taking an osteoporosis medicine.

What is Osteopenia?

"Osteopenia is the thinning of bone mass. While this decrease in bone mass is not usually considered 'severe', it is considered a very serious risk factor for the development of osteoporosis. Osteopenia is commonly seen in people over age 50 that have lower than average bone density but do not have osteoporosis. The diagnostic difference between the two is the measure of bone mineral density." (spine universe)

What is Osteoporosis?

"Osteoporosis, which literally means porous bone, is a disease in which the density and quality of bone are reduced. As bones become more porous and fragile, the risk of fracture is greatly increased. The loss of bone occurs silently and progressively. Often there are no symptoms until the first fracture occurs."
(iofbonehealth – what)

Not everyone will get Osteopenia or Osteoporosis. There are a few factors that may increase the chances: gender, race, family history, age, lifestyle choices, and other medical conditions. Even though it's not reversible, you can prevent it before it gets out of control or slow it down: a healthy diet, supplements if needed (calcium, magnesium, Vitamin D, K, & C), weight bearing exercises (jogging, walking, strength training), no smoking or excessive use of alcohol, regular check-ups, and bone health medications (Zometa).
(spineuniverse – conditions)

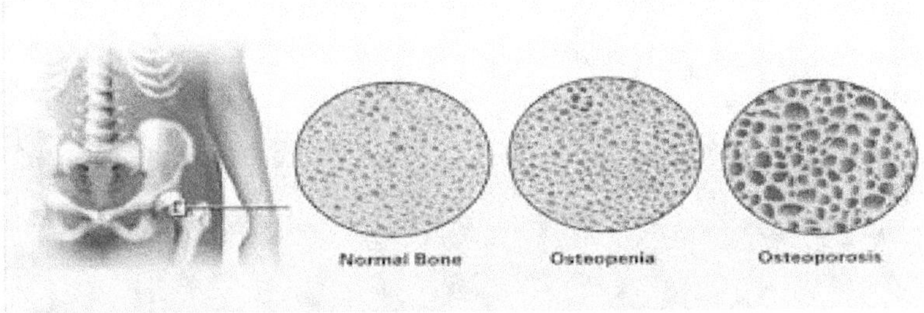

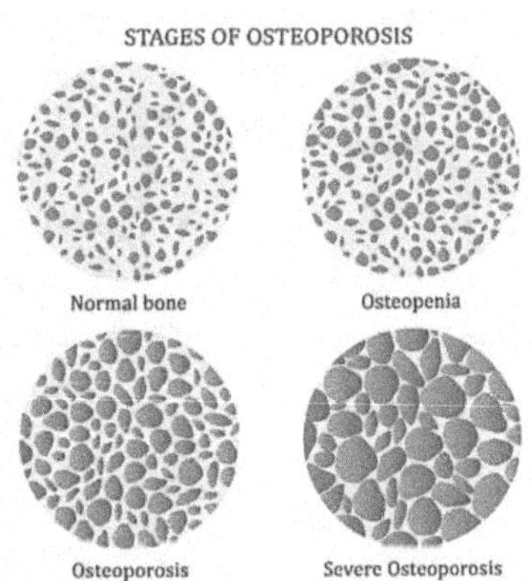

Day 1

Breakfast
8 oz. orange juice fortified with calcium and vitamin D
1 cup whole-grain cereal fortified with vitamin D
4 oz. skim milk

Lunch
2.5oz. Extra-lean ground beef on a whole-grain bun (may add 1 slice nonfat American cheese, 1 lettuce leaf, and 2 red tomato slices)
Green salad with 1 hard-boiled egg and 2 Tbsp. low-calorie dressing
8oz. Skim milk

Snack
1 orange

Dinner
2.5oz. Chicken breast
½ cup broccoli
¾ cup rice
2 slices French bread with 1 tsp. Margarine
1 cup strawberries with 2 Tbsp. lite whipped topping

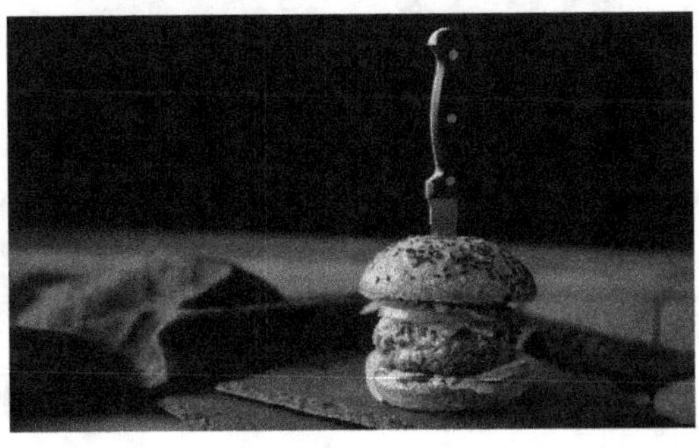

Day 2

Breakfast
1 slice whole-grain toast with peanut butter, avocado, or fruit jam
8 oz. calcium-fortified orange juice or 4 oz. skim milk

Lunch
Vegetarian chili
Green salad with 1 hard-boiled egg and 2 Tbsp. low-calorie dressing
Small serving sorbet with raspberries

Snack
Low or nonfat yogurt with sliced fruit or berries

Dinner
Pasta primavera with whole-grain pasta, grilled chicken, yellow
squash, zucchini, carrots, and cherry tomatoes, dressed in olive oil

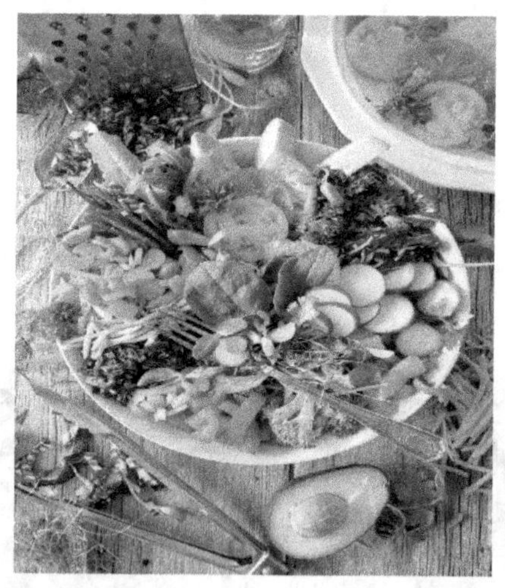

Day 3

Breakfast
Slow-cooked oatmeal prepared with apples and/or raisins
8 oz. calcium-fortified orange juice

Lunch
Falafel pita sandwich (may add cucumber, lettuce, and tomato)
1 slice watermelon

Snack
1 apple, banana, or orange, or 1 serving of strawberries

Dinner
Fajita burrito with chicken or lean steak, bell peppers, onions and
quinoa on a whole-grain tortilla
Mashed sweet potato
Corn

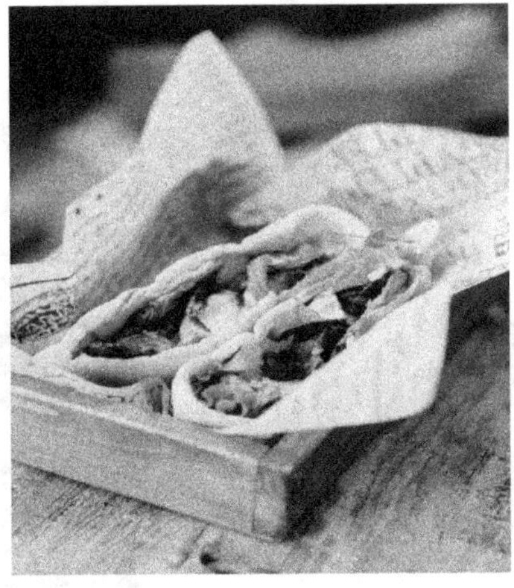

Day 4

Breakfast
Scrambled tofu with vegetables (bell peppers, sugar snap peas, spinach)
Oven-roasted potatoes (may sprinkle with skim-milk American shredded cheese)

Lunch
Whole-wheat wrap with red pepper hummus, grated carrots, and tomato (may also try black or white bean spreads)
1 apple or banana

Snack
Fruit smoothie blended with low-fat yogurt or skim milk

Dinner
Grilled chicken sautéed with zucchini, asparagus, and mushrooms
Corn on the cob

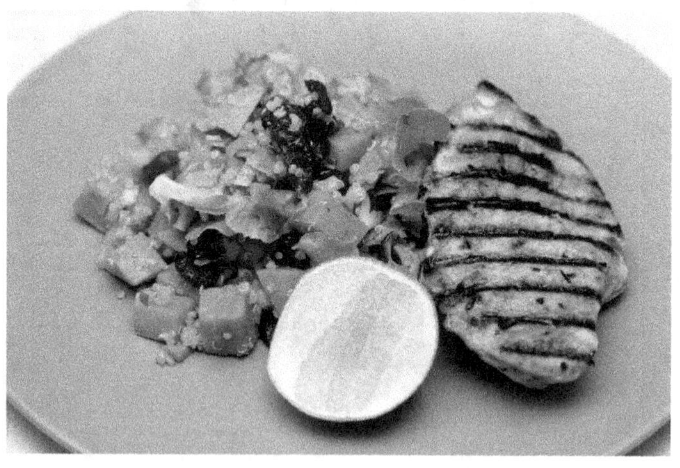

Day 5

Breakfast
Whole-grain cereal with sliced strawberries
4 oz. soy milk
1 small banana

Lunch
Thai soup with noodles, spinach mushrooms, and corn
Carrot and bean dip with celery and/or carrots for dipping
Snack
Chickpea or white bean dip
1 toasted whole-grain pita, sliced into fours for dipping

Dinner
Whole-grain spaghetti with vegetables (chopped onions, grated
carrots, diced broccoli)
Small serving sorbet with berry sauce or fruits

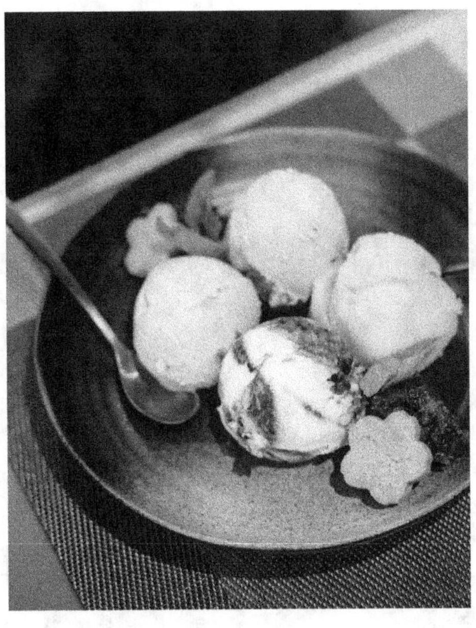

Day 6

Breakfast
Whole-grain pancakes topped with applesauce or fruit spread
1 small veggie sausage link
4 oz. milk or calcium-fortified orange juice

Lunch
Vegetable or bean based soup
Black bean and corn salad with red peppers
1 apple, banana, or orange

Snack
4 cubes of low-fat cheese
Whole-grain crackers or crisps

Dinner
Whole-wheat spinach lasagna with low-fat cheese
Green salad with vegetables of your choice

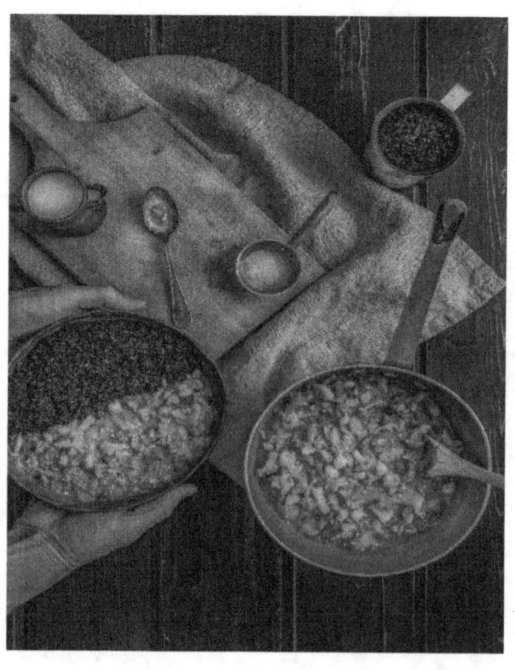

Day 7

Breakfast
Omelet or quiche with tomato, spinach, and other desired vegetables
8 oz. calcium-fortified juice or skim milk

Lunch
4- to 6- oz. salmon burger on a whole-grain bun
Mashed potatoes

Snack
Rice pudding or milk pudding prepared with low-fat milk
1 handful of unsalted almonds

Dinner
Nachos topped with kidney beans, avocado, and low-fat cheese
Greek salad with feta cheese

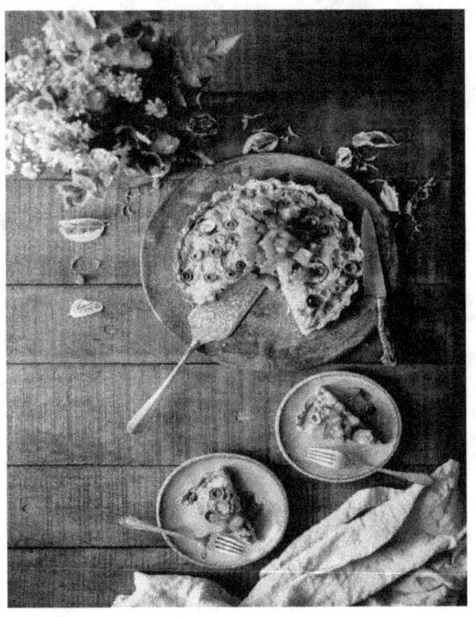

This meal plan was adopted from recommendations by the American Dietetic Association, the book "Building Bone Vitality: A Revolutionary Diet Plan to Prevent Bone Loss and Reverse Osteoporosis," and the International Osteoporosis Foundation, which offers many bone-friendly recipes.
More nutritious resources for bone health:
https://www.nof.org/patients/treatment/nutrition/

* Side note: The 7-day meal plan is just a guide to get you going. You can alter it any way you like based on your tastes, likes or dislikes. For me, I'd be pretty pleased with myself if I could maintain this daily. Honestly, I'm not in the kitchen enough or home enough or even get up early enough to make some of the breakfasts recommended!

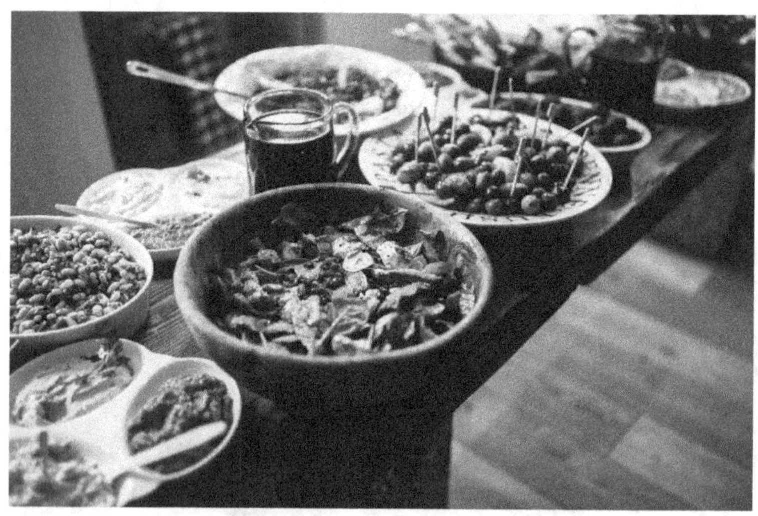

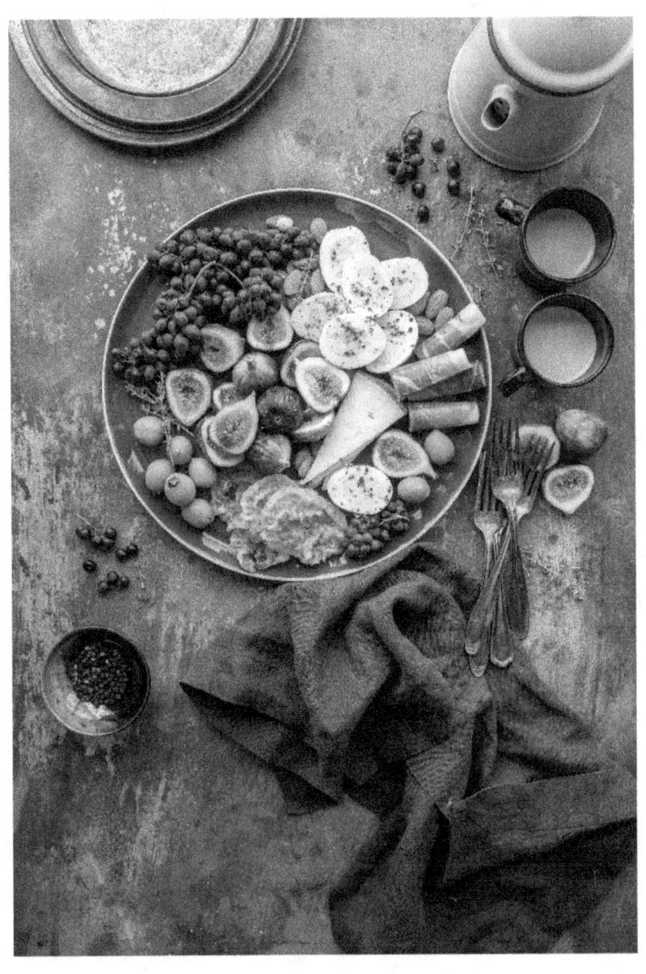

Supplements for Bone Health

Calcium

As we all know, calcium builds and keeps our bones healthy. Our bodies can't produce calcium, so it has to be provided through our food. If we don't get enough, then our body takes it from our bones. We need 1200mg daily (over 50 yrs.) and 1000mg daily (under 50). Although I'm under the age of 50, I still follow the protocol for over 50 and post-menopausal women. I just feel like the chemotherapy and the anti-hormone therapy has aged my body before it's time. Plus, I believe this is good preventive medicine to incorporate into my lifestyle sooner than later. This is the calcium supplement I take:

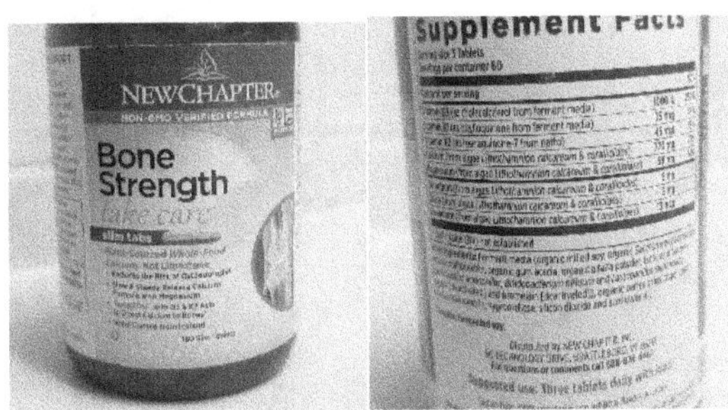

As you can see, this supplement includes Vitamin D3, Vitamin K1 & K2, Calcium and Magnesium. I only take this in the morning. The calcium content is listed at 770mg. In order to maintain the 1200mg needed for the day, I get the rest from food. This allows calcium intake and absorption throughout the day, and keeps me from relying solely on a supplement. Magnesium and zinc shouldn't be taken at the same time that calcium is taken because they compete for absorption with calcium losing out. This supplement includes Magnesium, but the milligrams are low. I take a higher magnesium dose in the evening as well as from food throughout the day.

Of course, dairy products are considered to have the highest in calcium, but there are many green vegetables that contain calcium as well. A lot of products are now fortified with calcium for our benefit; orange juice, bread, cereal to name a few.

Here are 15 calcium-rich foods per Healthline. I'm just going to list the food. I've provided a link to their site for more in-depth information.

- Seeds
- Cheese
- Yogurt
- Sardines & canned Salmon
- Beans & Lentils
- Almonds
- Whey Protein
- Leafy Greens
- Rhubarb
- Fortified Foods
- Amaranth
- Edamame & Tofu
- Fortified Drinks
- Figs
- Milk

(Healthline – calcium rich foods)

Calcium Calculator

To find out if you're getting enough calcium in your diet, you can calculate an estimated daily intake here. *The result of the calculation is an estimate and not an exact measure of calcium intake. Not all foods containing calcium are listed.* Check it out here: https://www.iofbonehealth.org/calcium-calculator

Magnesium

Magnesium converts vitamin D into the active form needed to promote calcium absorption. "An observational study of over 73,000 women found that those who consumed 400 mg of magnesium per day tended to have 2-3% higher bone density than women who consumed half this amount daily."
(Healthline – Magnesium)

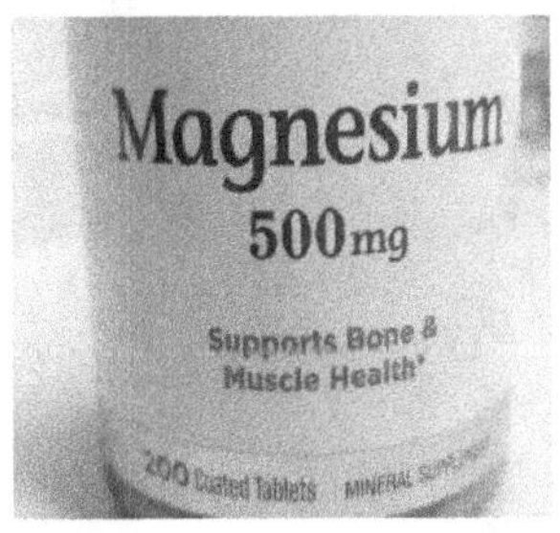

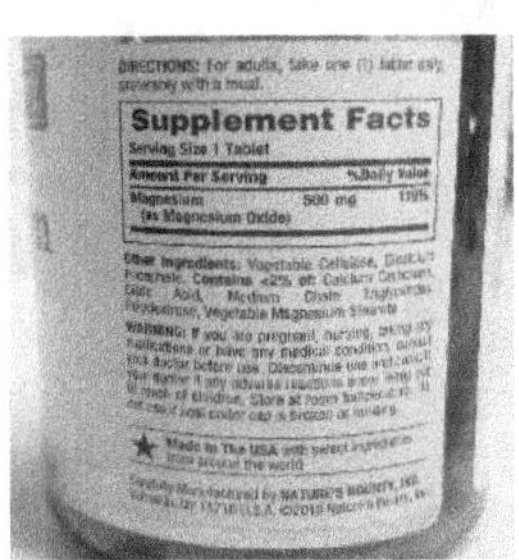

Women need 320mg daily. Men need 420mg. I know it looks like I'm taking a lot more than I need; 500mg before bed, and the 58mg that's included in my calcium supplement. My doctor had prescribed the extra magnesium during chemotherapy, and I maintained that for quite a while. I cut these in half; which gives me 250mg, plus the 58mg from the calcium supplement for a total of 308mg, then I get the rest from food.

With that being said, severe overdoses of magnesium are rare. "Occasionally, a high dosage of magnesium from supplements or medications can cause mild symptoms of an overdose, including diarrhea, nausea, and stomach cramps." (Magnesium - Medical News Today)

Here is a list of foods that are rich in magnesium to supplement your supplement!

-   Dark chocolate (Yay!)
-   Nuts
-   Seeds
-   Avocado
-   Legumes
-   Tofu
-   Fatty fish (salmon, tuna)
-   Banana
-   Cherries
-   Peaches
-   Blackberries
-   Figs
-   Green peppers
-   Spinach
-   Broccoli

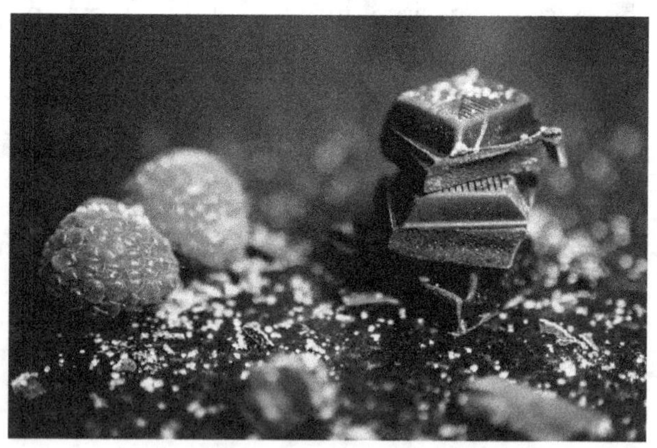

Zinc and copper are important trace minerals that are necessary in the growth and development of the skeletal system. Adequate levels of both are important to maintain to prevent or treat osteopenia or osteoporosis. These two minerals need to be balanced. Every 30mg of zinc needs to be balanced by 2mg of copper. "Recommended doses for the treatment and prevention of osteoporosis are 15mg to 30mg zinc and 1.5mg to 3mg copper a day." (Zinc Copper - Spine Universe)

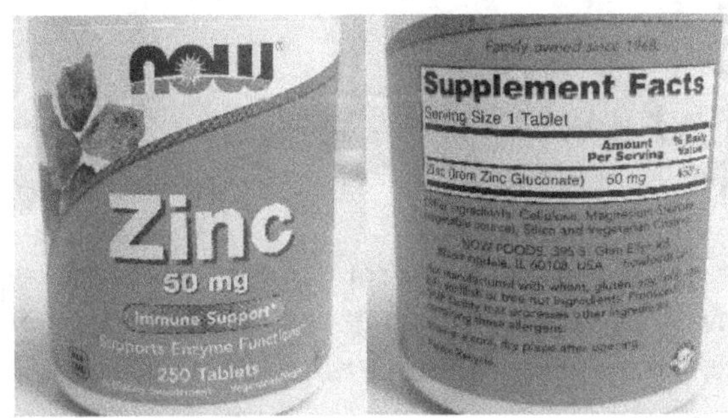

Foods that contain zinc:
- Beef
- Shrimp
- Spinach
- Flaxseeds
- Oysters
- Pumpkin seeds
- Pecans
- Oats

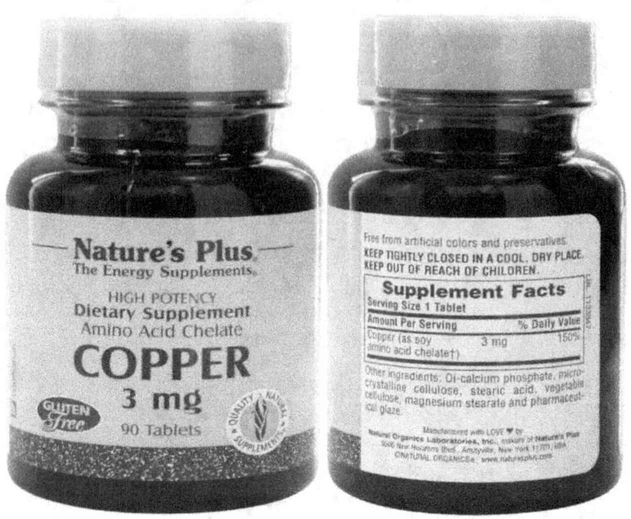

To comply with the zinc/copper ratio, I increased my copper intake from 2 to 3mg since I take 50mg of zinc. It's probably not necessary though. Here's another supplement that combines the two.

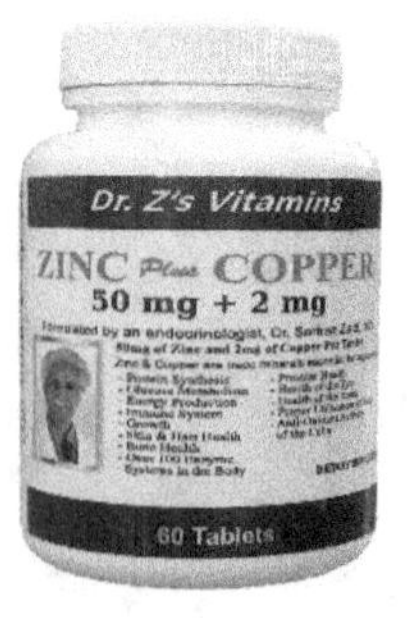

Each Tablet Contains:

50 MG OF ZINC
&
2 MG OF COPPER

Chelated with
Glycine for
Better Absorption

Supplement Facts

Serving Size 1 Tablet
Servings Per Container: 60

Amount Per Serving	%Daily Value	
Zinc (glycinate chelate)	50mg	333%
Copper (glycinate chelate)	2mg	100%

Other Ingredients: Dicalcium phosphate, vegetable stearic acid, croscarmellose sodium, vegetable magnesium stearate, silicon dioxide and aqueous film coating (purified water, hydroxypropyl methylcellulose, and vegetable glycerin).

ALLERGEN WARNING: CONTAINS SOY.

Foods that contain copper:
- Crab
- Buckwheat
- Liver
- Seeds & Nuts
- Mushrooms
- Peanut Butter

Vitamin D

Vitamin D helps your body absorb calcium. We need about 800-1000 IU daily (over 50yrs) and 400-800 IU daily (under 50 yrs.). (Vitamin D - nof.org)

- Sunshine
- Fatty fish (mackerel, salmon, tuna)
- Liver
- Cheese

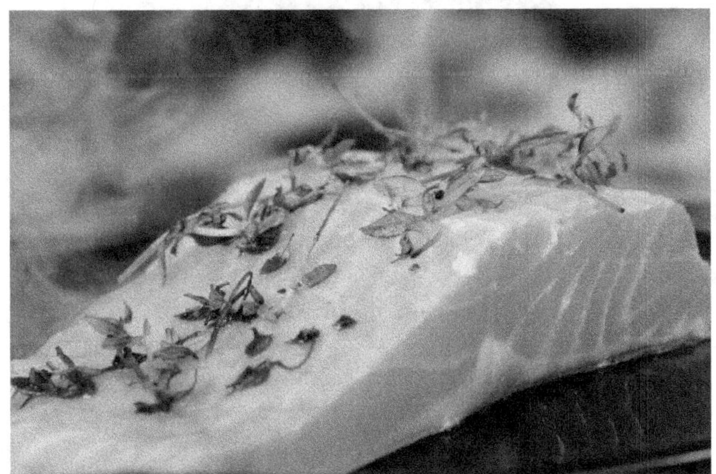

Vitamin C

Vitamin C is essential to the formation for collagen, the foundation that bone mineralization is built on. "It has recently been recognized as having an important role in the prevention and treatment of osteoporosis because of its ability to increase bone density. A typical dosage of Vitamin C is about 500mg to 1000mg per day." (Vitamin c - spine universe)
I take one every morning with my calcium supplement.

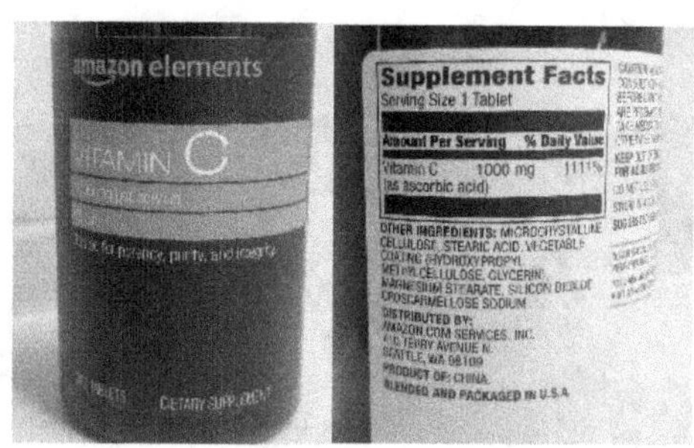

Foods that contain Vitamin C:
- Citrus (oranges, lemons, lime)
- Broccoli
- Green & red peppers
- Leafy greens
- Kiwi
- Strawberries
- Tomatoes
- Potatoes
- Cantaloupe

(AlgaeCal – vitamin c)

Vitamin A

"Vitamin A is a fat-soluble vitamin that is important to building strong healthy bones. Both osteoblasts (bone building cells) and osteoclasts (bone breaking down cells) are influenced by vitamin A. Despite its good effects, most clinical research links *higher* vitamin A levels with *lower* bone density and fractures."
(Vitamin A - American bone health)

Vitamin A can be found in:
- Red meat
- Fish
- Dark green vegetables
- Orange fruits.

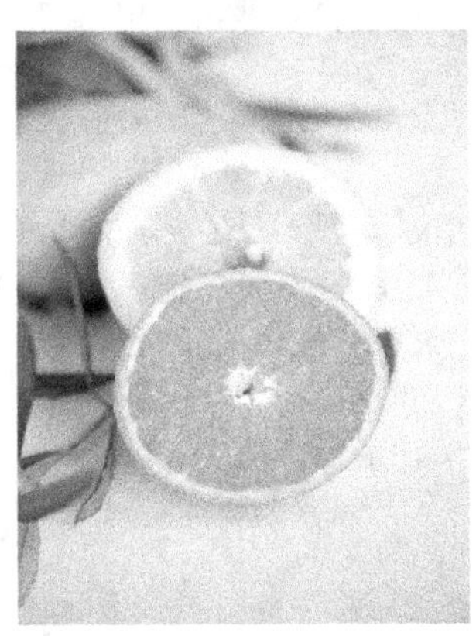

Vitamin K2
"Vitamin K2 supports bone health by modifying osteocalcin, a protein involved in bone formation. This modification enables osteocalcin to bind to minerals in bones and helps prevent the loss of calcium from bones. Studies have shown that vitamin K2 supports and increases bone density in postmenopausal women." (Vitamin K - Healthline)

Vitamin B12

"Low levels of vitamin B12 are linked to a higher risk of osteoporosis."
(Vitamin B12-American bone health)

Vitamin B12 can be found in:
- Dairy products
- Eggs
- Fish
- Poultry
- Supplements

Collagen
"Collagen is the main protein found in bones. It contains the amino acids glycine, proline and lysine, which help build bone, muscle, ligaments, and other tissues."
(Collagen-Healthline)

Omega-3 fatty acids
"The Omega-3s encourage the production of osteoblasts - the special cells that build bone."
Chia seeds/Flaxseeds
(Omega 3-AlgaeCal)

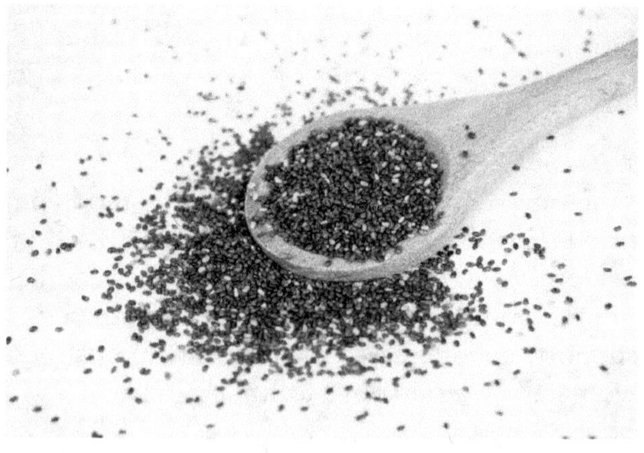

There has been controversy between scientists for decades on whether protein helps bone production or hinders it. This is most recent scientific research I found (feel free to correct me, if you find something even more recent):

"Recently, a series of investigations from various researchers and leading bone health societies including the International Osteoporosis Foundation (IOF), National Osteoporosis Foundation (NOF), American Bone Health, and American Society for Nutrition (ASN) have led to a clearer understanding of the role dietary protein plays in optimizing bone health across the life span. The IOF and European Society for Clinical and Economical Aspects of Osteoporosis, Osteoarthritis and Musculoskeletal Diseases now advise that dietary protein levels above the current RDA in the United States and Canada, regardless of the source, may be beneficial in reducing bone loss and hip fracture risk, provided calcium intakes are adequate. This article reviews the existing evidence to date and summarizes a recent webinar hosted by the ASN and American Bone Health in September of 2018.[12] Continuing Education credits for dietitians are available for viewing the on-demand webinar recording that can be found on the ASN website." (Protein-nutrition.org)

Exercises for muscle & bone health

Staying active reduces the risk of falls and fractures. It improves balance, strength, stamina and reduces pain. It's suggested to do weight bearing exercises for at least 30 minutes per day. If your feet hit the ground during exercise, it's more than likely weight bearing. Walking or jogging is considered weight bearing; swimming or biking are not.

Here are a few exercises that combine strength, balance and endurance:
- Strength training using your body weight
- Stretching
- Tai Chi
- Walking
- Low-impact dancing
- Low-impact aerobics
- Stair climbing

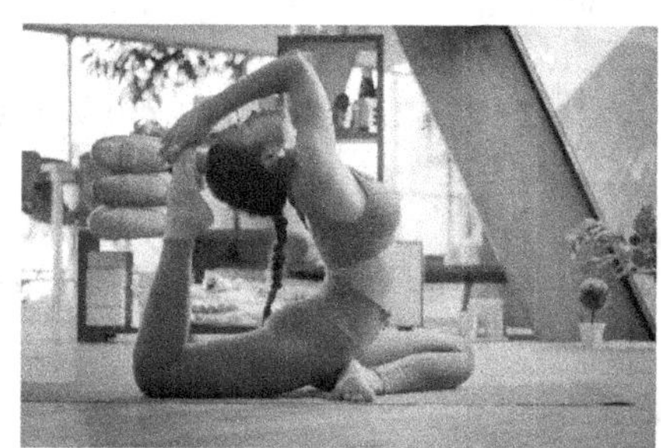

Exercises to *avoid* if you have Osteopenia or Osteoporosis

Your bone density score will determine how high a risk you are for fractures or broken bones. The overall recommendation is to avoid high-impact exercises such as jumping, or running. Other activities to avoid involve bending or twisting at the waist; touching your toes, sit-ups, golf, tennis, bowling, some yoga poses and some Pilates.

Medication for Bone health

Zometa *(zoledronic acid)*. Here's what I found: "Zometa is a bisphosphonate medicine that alters bone formation and breakdown in the body. This can slow bone loss and may help prevent bone fractures." (Medication – Zometa)

That sounds simple enough, but let's take a look at what www.breastcancer.org says about the same drug. "Bisphosphonates limit the activity of certain bone cells, called osteoclasts, which help cause the bone weakening and destruction that can happen *when breast cancer spreads to the bone.* Bisphosphonates also can help keep blood calcium levels normal - important because destruction of bone may increase blood calcium. Zometa is typically used to reduce bone complications and bone pain caused by *advanced-stage breast cancer* that has spread to the bone. It's usually given with other chemotherapy medicines." (Emphasis mine) (Medication – breast cancer)

The side effect list is long. Here are a few highlighted ones: depression, dizziness, irregular heartbeat, lethargy, nausea/vomiting, rapid weight gain (*great*), seizures, skin rash, and sore throat to name a few. (Medication-drugs.com-Zometa)

I was scheduled for an infusion of Zometa in September 2020. I read the long list of side effects, but my oncologist reassured me that because I'll only be getting this every six months, I should be fine. He briefly mentioned getting a dental appointment, sent me a list of dental clinics in the area, and put in a request to be seen at the Veteran's Affairs Dental clinic for a clearance. I didn't think anything about it, and honestly, kind of blew it off. I never made an appointment locally with a dentist and the VA never called to schedule a dental appointment with them either. In the meantime, I was preparing myself mentally for another infusion of chemicals that's supposed to help my health, despite all the nasty side effects. So, the day arrives and I go to my appointment with a focused mindset (it's just one more step… just one more step). My oncologist informs me that my infusion will be postponed until December 2020; a few days before Christmas (Merry Christmas to me). What? I feel instant relief, but curious and somewhat annoyed. He explains that the VA Dental clinic denied the appointment (I don't have a high enough disability to be seen there), and I haven't been cleared by a dentist to receive the medication. Osteonecrosis of the Jaw was briefly mentioned, but not entirely explained. He finished my examination, and I left completely dumbfounded.

A week later, the VA Dental clinic calls again to schedule a dental exam. Now, I'm confused. They explained that my oncologist had resubmitted the request for dental clearance along with the reasons for the exception. So, they schedule me for the appointment as well as a COVID-19 test two days prior. *Side note: I'm not sure how many of you have had a drive-thru COVID test, but it's not very pleasant! They slide that swab up your nostril and tickle your brain until your eyes water! Whew! I went to my dental appointment, and after x-rays, they were generous enough to give me a full cleaning. They scheduled me for Oral Surgery to pull a broken tooth, then cleared me for oncology and the Zometa. What a mess!

Guess what? My oncologist called me two days later to tell me that they misread my DEXA scan. My score is -1.4 not -1.9, so I don't need the Zometa. They canceled the drug and the infusion. At this point, I don't even know what to say.

What exactly is Osteonecrosis of the Jaw?

According to BreastCancer.org, "Osteonecrosis of the jaw is a *rare* but serious condition in which the cells in the jawbone start to die." This may be caused by bisphosphonates, medicines used to strengthen bones:
- Actonel (risedronate)
- Aredia (pamidronate disodium)
- Bonefos (clodronate)
- Boniva (ibandronate)
- Fosamax (alendronate sodium)
- Zometa (zoledronic acid)

"Researchers think that osteonecrosis of the jaw may develop because bisphosphonates stop the body from repairing microscopic damage to the jawbone. It's not clear why this happens in some people and not in others. Because some breast cancer treatments can cause bone loss (osteoporosis), many women being treated for breast cancer also take a bisphosphonate."

Symptoms include:
- Pain, swelling, redness, or other signs of infection in the gums
- Gum or sockets that don't heal after dental work
- Loose teeth
- Numbness or a heavy feeling in the jaw
- Draining
- Having bone become visible in your mouth

(Osteonecrosis – breastcancer.org)

The American Association of Oral and Maxillofacial Surgeons (AAOMS) concluded that risk in the overall cancer population *not* receiving bisphosphonates ranged from 0% to 0.019% (0-1.9 cases per 10,000 cancer patients). The study in breast cancer patients found that odds in patients treated with zoledronate (Zometa) increased threefold (3.23 or 95%)." In the final conclusion of the study, AAOMS concluded that "the risk of osteonecrosis among cancer patients exposed to zoledronate ranges between 50-100 times higher than cancer patients treated with a placebo." (Osteonecrosis – Medscape)

Isn't it amazing how one medication is good for one thing, but causes a multitude of problems somewhere else? Now I understand how some people end up taking over twenty different medications daily!

Pain Management (joint, back, bones)

When I take the proper dose of Letrozole, as prescribed by my doctor, the bone pain becomes severe enough to render me useless. My lower back and hips seem to suffer the most, with my knees and shoulders being a close second. Sometimes, I feel like I could benefit in using a walker. Other times, I'm crawling up the stairs. Pain has even awakened me in the middle of the night. I shuffle to the bathroom for ibuprofen. The frustrating part is that I'm only in my forties, but feel so much older. In cutting my pills in half, it seems as though the pain has been reduced, but not entirely eliminated.

So, what are the options for pain management?

A pain management clinic is where doctors offer solutions to intractable pain. Conditions that generally respond well to pain clinic services are arthritis, back pain and cancer. Migraine headaches, shingles pain, and carpal tunnel syndrome pain frequently respond favorably to pain clinic treatments.

Generally, pain management consists of a combination of treatments or therapies. These include medication, physical therapy and nerve blocks. They treat acute pain and perform diagnostics to determine the origin of the pain. A majority of pain management clinics focus on diagnosis and management of chronic pain. Some specialize in specific diagnosis and others specialize in pain related to a particular area of the body. Therapy plans are typically tailored to each individual's need, circumstance and preference.

Over-the-Counter (OTC) medication
- Tylenol
- NSAIDS (nonsteroidal anti-inflammatory drugs): ibuprofen (Motrin, Advil); naproxen (Aleve, Naprosyn) or diclofenac gel

Prescription medication https://drugs.com
Corticosteroids: reduces spontaneous discharge in an injured nerve
- Dexamethasone
- Prednisone
- Prednisolone

Opioids: often used to treat chronic pain or acute pain
- Hydrocodone (Vicodin)
- Oxycodone (OxyContin, Percocet)
- Morphine
- Codeine
- Fentanyl

Tricyclic Antidepressants: may increase neurotransmitters in the spinal cord that reduce pain signals. But they generally take several weeks to work.
- Amitriptyline
- Nortriptyline (Pamelor)
- Protriptylne (Vivactil)
- Doxepin (Silenor)
- Imipramine (Tofranil)
- Clomipramine (Anafranil)
- Desipramine (Norpramin)

Anticonvulsants (anti-seizure): this medication can be used for pain caused by nerve damage (neuropathy) which can be caused by many conditions; diabetes, shingles, chemotherapy, herniated disk, and others.
- Gralise
- Neurontin
- Horizant
- Pregabalin (Lyrica)
- Carbamazepine
- Oxcarbazepine
- Phenytoin (Dilantin)
- Lamotrigine (Lamictal)
- Valproic acid (Depakene)

Lidocaine patches: Used to relieve pain of postherpetic neuralgia, burning/stabbing pain or aches that last for months or years. It works by stopping nerves from sending pain signals.

Bone pain: aching or other discomfort in one or more bones
If pain is related to thinning bones, you may need treatment for osteoporosis.
<See Osteoporosis chapter>

Over-the-counter medication
- Tylenol
- NSAIDS (nonsteroidal anti-inflammatory drugs): ibuprofen (Motrin, Advil); naproxen (Aleve, Naprosyn) or diclofenac gel
- Sprays
- Creams

Muscle pain or myalgia: muscle pain can involve a small area or your whole body, ranging from mild to excruciating.

Utilize RICE:
- Rest: take a break from normal activities
- Ice: Place an ice pack on the sore area for 20 minutes throughout the day
- Compression: wrap in a compression bandage to reduce swelling
- Elevation: elevate to reduce swelling

Over-the-counter medication
- Tylenol
- NSAIDS (nonsteroidal anti-inflammatory drugs): ibuprofen (Motrin, Advil); naproxen (Aleve, Naprosyn) or diclofenac gel
- Sprays
- Creams

Muscle cramps: sudden, involuntary contractions that occur in various muscles. Dehydration can cause muscle cramps. Low levels of the following minerals can also cause cramping: calcium, potassium, sodium, and magnesium.

Utilize RICE:
- Rest: take a break from normal activities
- Ice: Place an ice pack on the sore area for 20 minutes throughout the day
- Compression: wrap in a compression bandage to reduce swelling
- Elevation: elevate to reduce swelling

Over-the-counter medication
- Tylenol
- NSAIDS (nonsteroidal anti-inflammatory drugs): ibuprofen (Motrin, Advil); naproxen (Aleve, Naprosyn) or diclofenac gel
- Sprays
- Creams

Arthritis/joint pain:
Exercising regularly may help decrease pain and increase mobility and flexibility without causing joint damage. Low-impact exercises or activities, ice packs, and OTC pain medications are recommended. Depending on the severity, RICE, creams, sprays, or massage therapy may be beneficial.

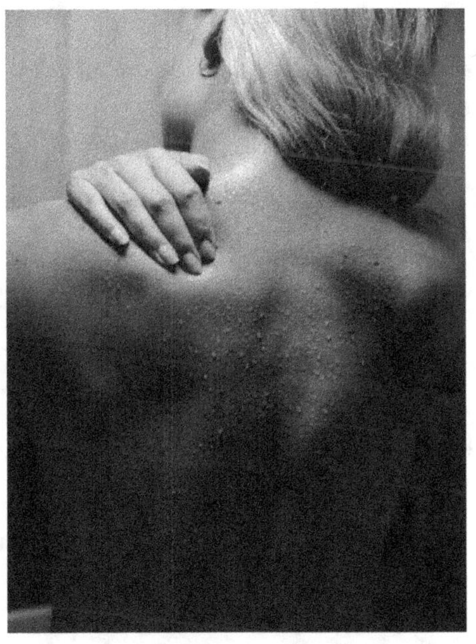

Fatigue

Sleep eludes me. 2.5mg of Letrozole makes it difficult to sleep completely through the night. Even with half a pill, sometimes it's still a struggle. I feel exhausted all the time. For me, taking this medication in the morning is disastrous. It's difficult to stay awake throughout the day; especially at work. At home, I sat down on the couch and was instantly asleep. At night? Intermittently.

I was on my way home from work one day and pulled over to the side of the road in a nearby neighborhood. I needed to send a text asking if I should stop the grocery store before going home. I put the car into PARK, sent the text, then fell asleep.

Another time, I was house/pet sitting for a friend. After work, I drove to her house, pulled into the driveway, put the car into PARK, and fell asleep. Sounds dangerous, doesn't it?

My solution… I now take my pill right before bed. I set an alarm and take it the same time every single night. Do I still have issues with sleeping through the night? Absolutely. But, I'm not randomly falling asleep during the day either.

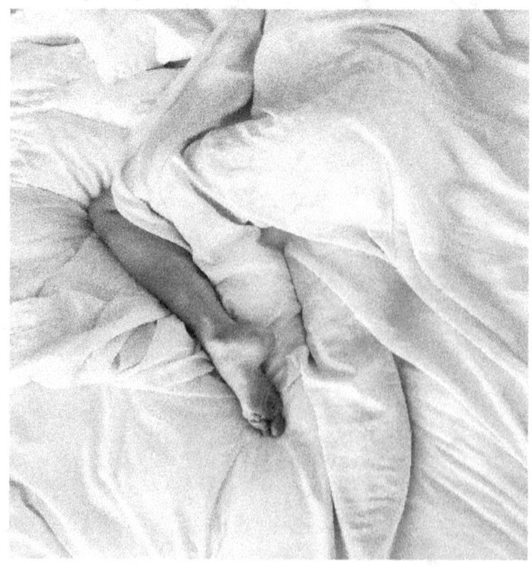

To sleep through the night:

OTC medication:
- Diphenhydramine (Benadryl, Aleve PM)
- Doxylamine succinate (Unisom Sleep Tabs)

Prescription medication: these are for short-term use only
- Benzodiazepines (Ativan, Valium, Klonopin, Restoril)
- Atypical benzodiazepines (Ambien, Sonata, Lunesta)
- Melatonin agonists (Rozerem)
- Antidepressants (Silenor, amitriptyline, trazodone)
- Suvorexant (Belsomra)

Natural remedy

"*Melatonin* helps regulate circadian rhythm and synchronize our sleep-wake cycle with night and day. In doing so, it facilitates a transition to sleep and promotes consistent, quality rest. Melatonin created within the body is known as endogenous melatonin, but the hormone can also be produced externally. Exogenous melatonin is made synthetically as a dietary supplement." (sleep foundation – melatonin)

Valerian is a sedating herb that is used to insomnia and anxiety. It's believed to work by increasing brain levels of the calming chemical GABA. This herb works best when taken daily for two or more weeks.

Chamomile has gentle sedative properties. To get the full sleep-promoting benefit, bring water to a boil, add 2-3 tea bags, cover with a lid, and brew for 10 minutes.

Chemo Brain/Brain Fog

Chemo brain or brain fog is truly frustrating!

Since the completion of chemotherapy, the fog is gradually starting to lift. But every now and then, I still have a moment. I don't know if it's a remnant from the chemo days, if it's caused by anti-hormone therapy or just the proverbial "getting older" syndrome.

According to MD Anderson, chemobrain is "a symptom reported by many cancer patients with difficulty processing information. It is a legitimate, diagnosable condition that can be caused by chemotherapy, the cancer itself, or a secondary medical condition."

Symptoms
- Difficulty concentrating on a single task
- Problems with short-term memory: forgetting details or recent events
- Feeling mentally "slower" than usual
- Confusing dates and appointments
- Misplacing objects
- Fumbling for the right word or phrase

Symptoms of chemo brain can fade after chemo treatment ends. Some may take a year or more; others may never regain full mental ability.

Interesting fact: Estrogen helps support certain types of brain functioning; cognition. The decrease in estrogen can cause occasional episodes of forgetfulness or "fuzzy brain".

Treatment

There really is no treatment for this. Some patients have found relief through stimulants like Ritalin. Ritalin, often used for ADHD, can help improve focus, concentration and stamina.

Other coping strategies
- Exercise: 5-10 minutes of mild to moderate exercise
- Memory aids: notebooks, planners, lists. This is what I use. I have notebooks, journals and planners all over the place. I find old-fashioned paper and pens are best for me, but do utilize technology as well. For example, I set an alarm on my phone to remind me to take my pills every night.
- Treat fatigue and sleep problems. These two issues can make chemo brain worse.
- Minimize distractions: a more sound-proof environment, like an office rather than a cubicle can decrease distractions and improve concentration.

**Interesting fact:* Employers are required by the American Disabilities Act to make reasonable accommodations for health-related issues.

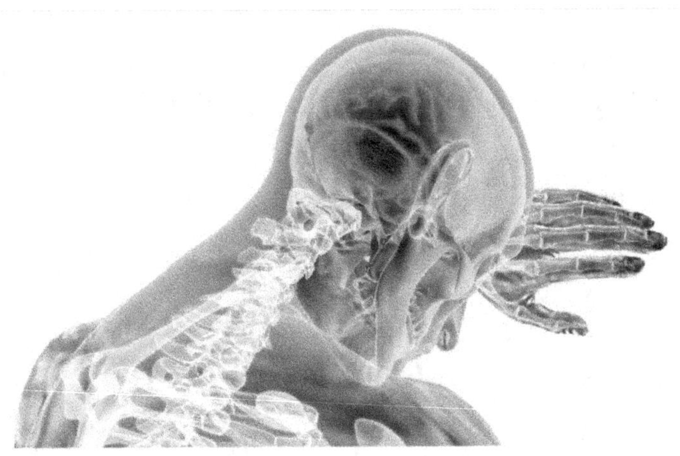

Mood Swings

I don't remember having any mood swings throughout this journey; cancer, chemo or anti-hormone therapy. But! I'm sure the people around me would probably tell you differently. We all know how emotional this experience can be, so with that being said, mood swings are bound to happen!

Although mood can be affected by multiple things, from arguments to traffic jams, "it's not always clear as to what causes mood swings and the irritability that often accompanies them." <Healthline>

Estrogen regulates several hormones that may boost the mood: serotonin, norepinephrine, and dopamine. With the decrease in estrogen comes forgetfulness and a "fuzzy brain"; which, leads to frustration and a bad mood. Not all women will have mood swings. There's no formula for who will experience them or who won't.

Ideas to reduce or diminish mood swings
- Exercise
- Healthy eating
- De-stress
- Plenty of sleep

When mood swings become extreme, cause additional anxiety, or it becomes difficult to participate in life, then it's time to chat with your doctor.

Prescriptions
My rule of thumb is to try everything before resorting to medical prescriptions. Sometimes, there is no other alternative. Treatment and therapy usually involves a combination of medications and psychotherapy or counseling. In looking for prescription mood stabilizers, my search brought up a multitude of psychiatric disorders. I'm only looking at hormonal mood swings. If you feel you're beyond the hormonal mood swing, by all means talk to a doctor.

Mood stabilizers
- Valproic acid (Valproic)
- Lamotrigine (Lamictal)
- Oxcarbazepine (Trileptal)

Natural Remedies:
- St. John's Wort is good alternative for managing depression
- Vitamin D has also been proven to moderate mood
- Light therapy (more on this in a later chapter)
- Acupuncture
- Yoga

Hot Flashes

UGH. What more can I say? An internal inferno super power that can fog up glasses, melt snow, and fry eggs. It can also leave you soaked, make you strip unsexily, and stand inside the freezer.

As you know, hot flashes or night sweats are a common symptom for menopause that can last for many years. Because most of us are taking anti-hormone medication, this symptom could be more extreme or prolonged. Before turning to medication, let's explore a few options to help manage those hot flashes. Besides, our options for prescription medication is limited due to our anti-estrogen predicament.

I personally keep my bedroom cooler at night; ceiling fan, additional window A/C unit despite the house already having A/C and ice water on the nightstand.
- Dress in layers
- Portable fan
- Avoid alcohol, spicy food, caffeine, and smoking
- Maintain a healthy weight (not always very easy)
- Self-calming techniques: mindfulness, meditation, yoga, tai chi

Non-hormone option: Paroxetine - a low-dose selective serotonin reuptake inhibitor (SSRI) antidepressant.
The side effects include dizziness, headache, nausea, jitteriness, and possibly drowsiness.

Natural Remedy:
Unfortunately for us breast cancer survivors, most of these herbal supplements are off limits or not recommended. If you read the previous discussion on estrogen, you'll find all the information. What a bummer!

I've listed the following are herbs that improve women's health and menopause, what they've been used for in the past as well as today. The efficacy for treating menopausal symptoms, the active ingredients and the effects on human physiology is still unknown. Use caution.

Black Cohosh: Native Americans used this to treat musculoskeletal pain, fever, cough, pneumonia, sluggish labor, and menstrual irregularities. Today, this herb is used mostly for menopausal symptoms; hot flashes, night sweats, vaginal dryness, heart palpitations, tinnitus, vertigo, sleep disturbances, nervousness and irritability. (Hot flashes – black cohosh)

Red Clover: Historically, this herb was used for asthma, whooping cough, cancer and gout. Today, Isoflavones extracts from red clover are used as dietary supplements for menopausal symptoms, high cholesterol and osteoporosis. (Hot flashes – red clover)

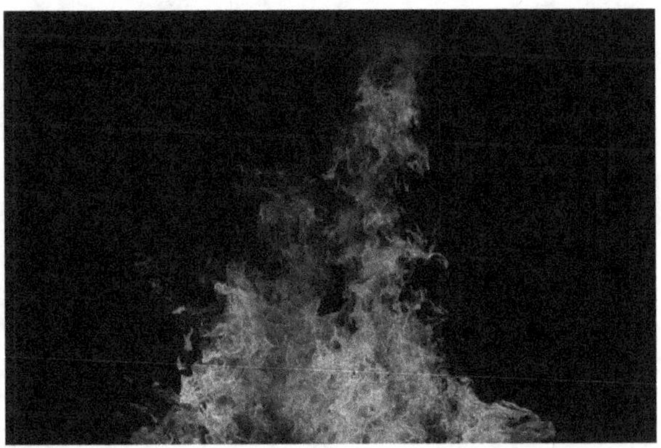

Dong Quai: This herb has been used as an herbal medicine for more than 2,000 years. It's used to build blood health, boost or activate blood circulation, treat blood deficiency, regulate the immune system, relieve pain, relax the bowels, treat premenstrual syndrome, and to relieve symptoms of menopause.
(Hot flashes – dong quai)

Siberian Ginseng: This herb has been used for centuries, specifically in China and Russia. It was traditionally used to prevent colds and flu, to increase energy, longevity and vitality. It's widely used in Russia as an "adaptogen"; a substance that is supposed to help the body better cope with either mental or physical stress. Today, it's also used to reduce chemotherapy side effects, stimulate the immune system, to increase strength and stamina, to reduce osteoarthritis symptoms, and to improve bone metabolism in post-menopausal women. (Hot flashes – Siberian ginseng)

Kava: "The active compounds in kava (kavalactones) provide pain relief and act as muscle relaxants and anticonvulsants. It may be effective in reducing anxiety and stress, but *liver toxicity and damage outweighs the benefits.*" (Hot flashes – kava)

Nausea/Vomiting

I haven't really had a lot of issues with nausea or vomiting from Letrozole. I might have vomited once or twice during chemo, but nothing more. I was prescribed a medication for nausea, but never really used it.

Here are a few tips on managing nausea:
Eat small amounts of food throughout the day
Eat dry foods: crackers, toast, cereal
Stay away from greasy foods
Take ginger or consume food with ginger in it
Don't lie down after eating
Request anti-nausea medication from your doctor
Holistic treatments: acupuncture, meditation, mindful eating

If you're vomiting often, try small sips of water or flat ginger ale and avoid eating for 4-8 hours. It's important to stay hydrated, so sipping broth, water, or juice is recommended. Apparently, the body will eventually get used to the anti-hormone medication and the nausea or vomiting will subside.

Diarrhea/Constipation

We've all had one or the other at some point in our lives. Sometimes, it's caused by a virus, food poison, or an unhealthy diet. For most of us reading this book, we can also include cancer, chemotherapy, and anti-hormone therapy.

Diarrhea
Self-treatment includes rehydration to prevent dehydration. Over-the-Counter anti-diarrheal medications such as Pepto-Bismol or Kaopectate can be very helpful.

For those that prefer something more natural, I recommend the BRAT diet which consists of Bananas, Rice, Applesauce and Toast. This diet is bland, starchy and low fiber that creates a binding effect to make loose stools bulkier.

Constipation
If you have less than three bowel movements per week, it's safe to say that you're constipated. Mild cases of constipation can be self-treated using over-the-counter medications (laxatives). Before now, I didn't know there were several different types of laxatives, and each one works differently.

Bulk-forming laxatives pull fluid into the intestines to make the stool softer and bulkier. This also produces intestinal muscle contractions that push the stool through the system. Drink lots of water when taking this type of laxative. This laxative may cause bloating or abdominal pain.

Lubricants coat the stool for easy passage through the intestine. This laxative starts working within 6-8 hours. This also may cause the body to absorb less of any medications or vitamins that you take regularly. It's not advisable to take this particular laxative long-term.

Osmotic laxatives help keep water inside the intestines, and usually act very quickly. Drink plenty of water to avoid dehydration when taking these. Osmotic laxatives can cause stomach cramping or diarrhea.

Stimulant laxatives cause intestinal contraction to move the stool through the system. These work within 6-10 hours after taking them.

It's not advisable to take this laxative long-term. Stomach cramping is the biggest side effect.

Stool softeners create softer bowel movements by adding water and fats to the stool. These usually take 1-3 days to take effect. There are very few side effects and relatively safe for long-term use.

Type	Generic and brand names	Forms	How fast?	Safe to use long-term?	Available as a generic?
bulk-forming	psyllium (Metamucil, Konsyl), calcium polycarbophil (FiberCon), methylcellulose fiber (Citrucel)	powder, granules, liquid, tablet, packet, wafer	a few days	yes	yes
lubricant	mineral oil (Fleet Mineral Oil Enema)	enema, oral liquid	6 to 8 hours	no	yes
osmotic	magnesium hydroxide (Phillips Milk of Magnesia), magnesium citrate, polyethylene glycol (Miralax), sodium phosphate (Fleet Saline Enema), glycerin (Fleet Glycerin Suppository)	enema, suppository, oral liquid	30 minutes or less	yes	yes
stimulant	bisacodyl (Dulcolax), senna/sennoside (Senokot)	enema, suppository, oral liquid or capsule	6 to 10 hours	no	yes
stool softener	docusate (Colace, DulcoEase, Surfak)	Enema, suppository, oral tablet, capsule, or liquid	1 to 3 days	yes	yes

(Healthline – constipation)

Prescription medications

Generic name	Brand name	Forms	How fast?	Safe to use long-term?	Available as a generic?
linaclotide	Linzess	oral capsule	within 24 hours for most people	yes	no
plecanatide	Trulance	oral tablet	within 24 hours for most people	yes	no
lubiprostone	Amitiza	oral capsule	within 24 hours for most people	yes	no
methylnaltrexone	Relistor	oral tablet, injection	within 24 hours for most people	yes	no
naloxegol	Movantik	oral tablet	within 24 hours for most people	yes	no

(Healthline – constipation prescription)

Natural remedies
Drink plenty of water. Dehydration can cause constipation. Sparkling water may even be more effective in relieving constipation.

Eat more soluble, non-fermentable fiber. Doctors always tell us to increase our fiber when dealing with constipation. Now there are new studies that suggest that increasing fiber can actually make the problem worse.

Fiber

There are two types of fiber, and each one has a different effect on the digestive system: soluble and insoluble fibers.
Soluble fibers: found in oat bran, barley, nuts, seeds, beans, lentils, peas as well as some fruits & vegetables. This absorbs water and creates a gel-like paste in the digestive tract, softening stools and improving consistency.

Insoluble fibers: found in wheat bran, vegetables, and whole grains. This fiber adds bulk to stools to help ease the passage through the digestive tract.

Now we have non-fermentable soluble fiber: psyllium. Psyllium is made from the husks of the Plantago ovata plant's seeds, also known as ispaghula. This is also beneficial for heart health, possible weight loss, pancreas, and diabetes.

Exercise. Gentle to moderate forms of exercise is thought to improve the digestive system; brisk walking, swimming, cycling. For some, vigorous exercise (running, jogging) could make symptoms worse.
Drink coffee. The caffeine in coffee stimulates the muscles in the digestive system the same way a meal does; which helps relieve constipation.

Senna is an herbal laxative. This is available in pill, suppository, or the natural herbal form for tea. Senna contains plant compounds called glycosides. These stimulate the nerves in the intestinal tract to speed up bowel movement. Recommended for short term use only.

Prebiotics are an indigestible carbohydrate fiber that improves digestive health by feeding the beneficial bacteria in the gut. This boosts the probiotics and improves overall balance of all gut bacteria. Foods include: chicory, artichokes, garlic, onions, bananas, leeks, and chickpeas.

Probiotics are beneficial bacteria that live in the digestive system. Maintaining probiotic balance can treat and prevent constipation. Foods include: yogurt, sauerkraut, and kimchi. Supplements are also available:

Glucomannan is a soluble fiber from the roots of the konjac plant. You can get this from shirataki noodles or by supplement. This supplement can help regulate bowel movements and prevent constipation. It's also added to various food products as a thickener in pasta and flour. I've used it to thicken up sauces. It can also cause a modest weight loss (more on that in subsequent chapters).

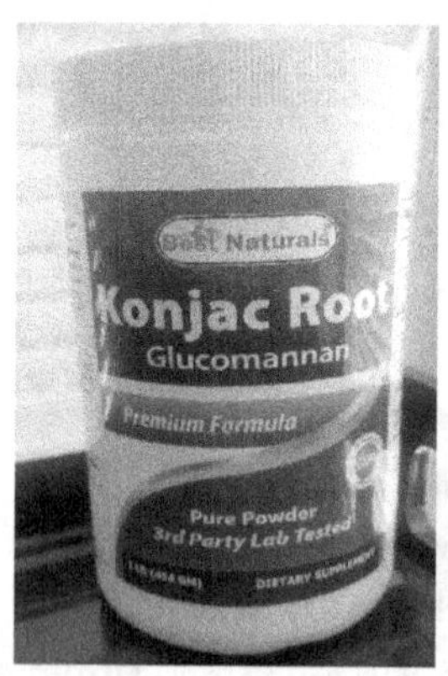

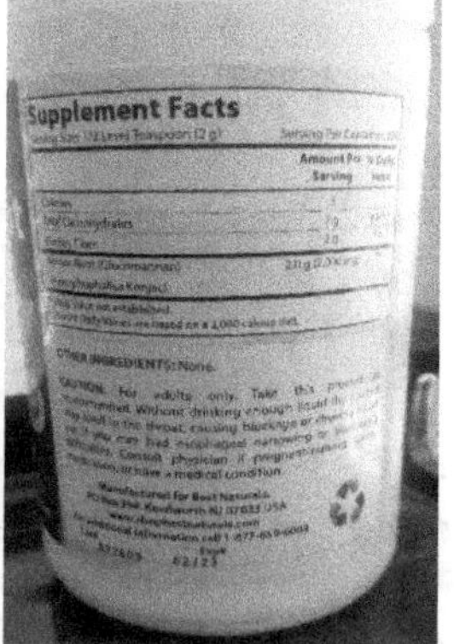

Vaginal dryness and other issues

"The decrease in estrogen with menopause is a major contributor to vaginal dryness, itching, burning, discomfort and pain during intercourse or other sexual activity. Vaginal atrophy may significantly affect your quality of life, sexual satisfaction, and relationship with your partner. Unlike hot flashes that improve with time, vaginal symptoms typically worsen with time because of aging and a prolonged lack of estrogen."

<u>*Non-Hormonal remedies*</u>

Vaginal lubricants
- water based options - Astroglide, K-Y Jelly, Doc Johnson GoodHead, Isabel Fay, Carrageenan
- All natural lubricants have a shorter shelf life - Aloe Cadabra, Sliquid Organics, Good Clean Love Almost Naked, Blossom Organics

Vaginal moisturizers can help prevent general itching and irritation, but don't provide enough wetness to prevent discomfort during penetration
Regular sexual stimulation

Vaginal dilators: "dilators are tube-shaped devices designed to help relax and lengthen the vagina, restore vaginal capacity and allow for more comfortable sexual activity. They're often confused with vibrators or dildos, but they are not sex toys. Dilator therapy is commonly prescribed to help heal pelvic pain in women's health."

Pelvic floor exercises: pelvic muscle training or Kegels is the practice of contracting and relaxing your pelvic floor muscles.

Vaginal Estrogen Therapy: I know what you're thinking… I was thinking about it too. Just hear me out…

"An effective and safe treatment, low-dose local estrogen is applied directly to the vagina to restore vaginal health and relieve vaginal dryness and discomfort with sexual activity. Improvements usually occur within a few weeks, although complete relief may take several months. *This may even be an option for women with a history of breast or uterine cancer but only after careful consideration of risk and benefits with a healthcare provider and oncologist.*" (emphasis mine)

It's definitely something to talk to your doctor about. The worst he could say is, "No".

Other prescription therapies:
- Ospemifene: an oral tablet taken daily for the treatment of painful intercourse caused by vaginal atrophy.
- Dehydroepiandrosterone (DHEA): a hormone containing insert placed in the vagina nightly for the treatment of painful intercourse caused by vaginal atrophy.

www.menopause.org The North American Menopause Society

Skin & Hair Changes

Menopause or medically induced menopause can bring some noticeable changes to the skin and hair. As hormone levels drop, skin can become dry, slack, and thin. There may also be more hair on your face than on your head!

To protect your skin:

- Apply sunscreen every day before going outdoors: this can help fade age spots, prevent new ones, and reduce skin cancer risk

- See a dermatologist for a skin cancer screening: the risk of skin cancer increases with age. The earlier you find it, the more treatable it is.

- Start skin self-exams: ask your dermatologist how and how often

- Treatment for age spots: ask your dermatologist for a skin exam; they can recommend an age-spot treatment that's perfect for your skin type.

"Skin cancer sometimes looks like an age spot or other dark spot on your skin. If you use your age-spot treatment on a skin cancer, you may fade the spot and delay treatment. Delaying treatment for skin cancer gives the cancer time to possibly grow and spread. This can make the cancer more difficult to treat."
(aad.org – skincare)

Bruising:

- Thin skin bruises easily. You may be able to reduce thinning skin.
- Apply a broad-spectrum sunscreen with SPF 30 or higher every day. This can actually prevent further thinning. You'll want to do this every day; even in the winter.
- Consult with a dermatologist; a retinoid cream may be more beneficial

Dry skin:

- Wash with a mild cleanser instead of soap.
- Apply moisturizer throughout the day.

Wrinkles:

After menopause, our skin loses collagen very quickly. As collagen diminishes, our skin loses its firmness and begins to sag. Permanent lines refuse to go away. Wrinkles are visible all the time. Pouches may form under your eyes. Ugh!

Again… the answer is protection from the sun. We also look for wrinkle remedies every chance we get and will pay top dollar, praying something will work.

Pimples/Acne:

Some women may develop teenage-like acne before or during menopause. But because our skin becomes thinner and drier, treatments for teenage acne can be too harsh.

- Wash with a cleanser that contains salicylic acid
- Avoid products that dry the skin
- If all fails, contact your dermatologist.

Hair treatment:

Due to the lowered production of estrogen and progesterone, some women will notice their hair thinning or their hairline is receding. The earlier you start treatment, the better the results. Hair loss can make you feel self-conscious, but the condition isn't permanent. Here are a few tip to keep your hair healthy:
- Reduce stress
- Exercise
- Eat healthy: green tea, vitamin B6 and folic acid help in restoring hair growth; fatty acids also play an important role in maintaining healthy hair- you'll find it in these foods: salmon, tuna, flaxseed oil, walnuts, almonds
- Hydrate
- Stay natural: stay away from heat tools (curling irons, dryers, straightening irons) to prevent drying and breakage. Extensions, dyes, perms compromise your scalp and hair health.

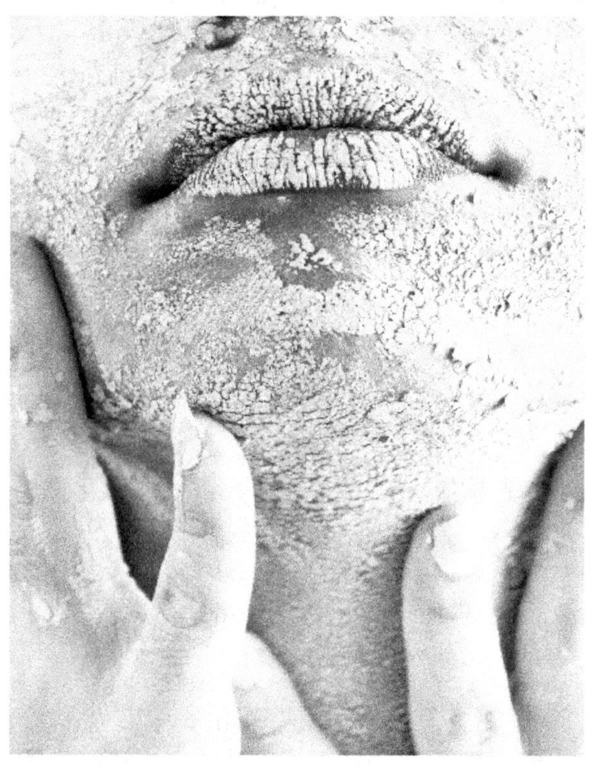

Weight Gain/Obesity

The only thing I was looking forward to when chemotherapy started was shedding a few pounds. Now, when I look at the girl *before* cancer and chemo, I think about how good she looked and how I'd give anything to look like that again. I think this is the hardest side effect to deal with for us women. Why is that? Is it the pressure of what society expects of women? Is it because we don't feel sexy with a few extra pounds? Or is it because we know it's unhealthy and could easily cause additional problems? Maybe it's a combination of all of those and more.

Here are a couple of pictures of me before cancer and after cancer.

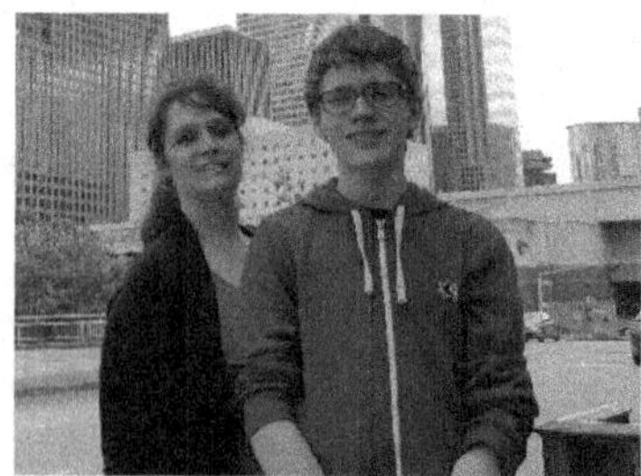

Before chemo (169 lbs.)

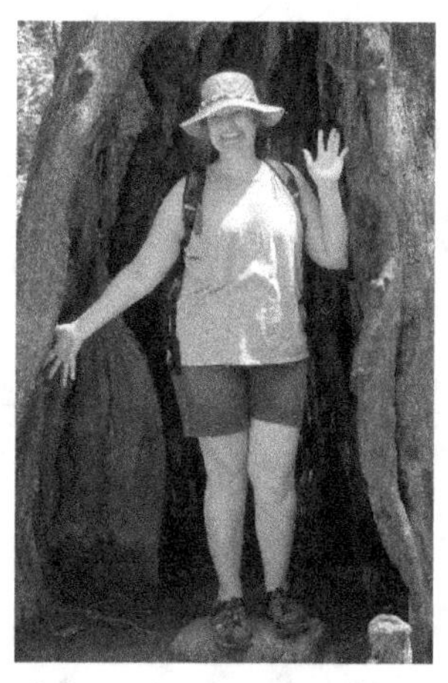

After chemo (200 lbs.)

Amazing, isn't it? And it's still a struggle to bring the weight down.

Here's a small slice of research that I found that actually explains what's going on inside the body:

"Many people gain weight when they are treated with chemotherapy and steroids. Your extra weight may hang around and increase after chemotherapy if you also take hormonal therapy (tamoxifen or an aromatase inhibitor). If your body shifts into menopause because of chemotherapy, there's a tendency to gain weight.
This weight gain may be because of the enzyme lipoprotein lipase (LPL), which is controlled by insulin. When lipoprotein lipase breaks down triglycerides, the fat molecules are used by the body as energy or stored in fatty tissue for later use. So basically, LPL sits on the surface of cells and pulls fat out of the bloodstream and into the cell. If LPL is on a muscle cell, it pulls fat into the cell where it's used for fuel. If LPL is on a fat cell, it pulls fat into the cell and makes it fatter.
It's important to know that the hormone estrogen suppresses LPL activity on fat cells. This could be one reason why some women gain weight after menopause or after breast cancer treatment that dramatically decreases estrogen levels. With less estrogen in the body, LPL can pull fat into fat cells and store it there." (Weight Gain – breast cancer tips)

How do you battle that??

Part 3: Rebuild

A Natural Remedy?

To find a natural replacement for anti-hormone therapy, I had to turn to Men's Health. There are men that have high levels of estrogen. This can cause several symptoms: the development of breast tissue, infertility, and erectile dysfunction. So, what are *they* doing to prevent this? And why can't we do the same?

As men age, their testosterone levels may drop. Those who experience low testosterone may also have elevated levels of estrogen. According to the Journal of Medicinal Food, estrogen-blocking foods that contain phytochemicals can help reduce estrogen levels in the bloodstream.

The following foods have a high level of phytochemicals that block estrogen production:

Cruciferous vegetables have a high level of phytochemicals and can be cooked in many different ways.
- Broccoli
- Cauliflower
- Cabbage
- Brussel sprouts
- Bok choy
- Kale
- Collard greens
- Turnips
- Rutabagas
- *Mushrooms* have been known to prevent the production of aromatase; which, is responsible for converting the hormone androgen over to estrogen.
- Shiitake
- Portobello
- Crimini
- Baby button

Red grapes
The skin of red grapes contain a chemical called resveratrol and the seeds contain a chemical called proanthocyanidin; both block estrogen production.

Seeds contain micronutrients called polyphenols.
- Flax seed contains some of the highest levels of polyphenols. They are also considered one of the richest sources of lignans, which act as phytoestrogens.
- Sesame seeds

Whole Grains, like seeds, contain anti-estrogen polyphenols and phytoestrogen nutrients, so an individual's response varies.
- Wheat
- Oats
- Rye
- Corn
- Rice
- Millet
- Barley

Green Tea is also a great source of polyphenols, which may influence enzymes that metabolize estrogens.

Pomegranates
This particular fruit is high in phytochemicals and is becoming widely known for their estrogen-blocking properties and their antioxidant virtues.

Natural Products as Aromatase Inhibitors

Wild Nettle Root
This herb is used to make medicine for the prostate. Nettle root contains substances that block testosterone conversion into estrogen. It's very useful in patients with estrogen dominance.

Chrysin
"This flavonoid is found in passionflower, honey and bee propolis. It's been argued that it blocks estrogen and increases testosterone; others claim there's no evidence.

Maca
This is considered a cruciferous plant that has many health benefits to include fertility. It supposedly has an anti-estrogen potential by reducing the conversion of testosterone.

Grape Seed Extract
This extract acts as an aromatase inhibitor in postmenopausal women with a high risk for breast cancer, but also works for men with an estrogen dominance.

Saw Palmetto
This is one of the most important herbs for men. The berries of this plant have been known to improve prostate health, balance hormone levels (to include estrogen), prevent hair loss, decrease inflammation and improve urinary function.
(Healthline – Saw Palmetto benefits)

CBD (Cannabidiol)/Medical Marijuana

I found loads of information on this topic. There are websites that claim that Cannabis as a whole cures cancer, while others claim it doesn't. Some say CBD oil may cause prescription medication to become more potent. Although it may not cure cancer, or replace hormone blockers or aromatase inhibitors, it can be used to manage the side effects. There is "anecdotal evidence that marijuana may ease pain, nausea/vomiting, hot flashes, loss of appetite, anxiety and insomnia." Pretty much everything I discussed in Part II. Just be honest with your doctor and treat it like any other drug. It may have the "potential for side effects, interactions with other drugs, as well as benefits." (CBD – breastcancer treatment) For those of you that have access to cannabis legally, I would recommend going to an actual medical marijuana clinic, rather than a shop that sells for recreational use.

What to Expect

"Medical marijuana comes in a variety of strains and each has different levels of active compounds and potency. The effects will be unique to each person and can be hard to predict. Again, because research on medical marijuana and cancer is limited, information on side effects is also limited. Reported side effects of medical marijuana include increased heart rate, low blood pressure, dizziness, fainting, hallucinations, and paranoia." (CBD – breastcancer treatment)

*Always tell your doctor about any vitamins, supplements, herbs and over-the-counter medicines you're using, including medical marijuana.

I used CBD oil and medical marijuana during my chemo treatments. I didn't take it every night, and only used it when I felt I really needed it. Some products were more potent than others, and some I wasn't sure if they did anything at all. My recommendation is to be smart about it, and do your research before moving forward with it. I don't use it anymore. I haven't really felt the need to.

Light Therapy

I first discovered light therapy while in Los Angeles, CA. There was a therapist administering light through a machine with pads to a cancer patient. Each pad had a multitude of red LED lights. I was intrigued, and started researching. At the time, it was very difficult to find a whole lot of information about this. I eventually found an online light therapy course, and decided to become a therapist. So what is light therapy?

"LED (light emitting diodes) therapy systems administer a combination of red, blue and infrared light to the skin, muscles, joints and bones. These wavelengths stimulate circulation and reduce pain. The lights are able to stimulate energy production, and penetrate surface tissue where they are absorbed by the underlying cells' mitochondria (a component within cells that involve energy production). Light therapy can provide temporary relief of minor pain, stiffness, and muscle spasms. It also increases local blood circulation which delivers more oxygen to the sites of treatment to speed up healing." (The Quantum Academies, 2013)

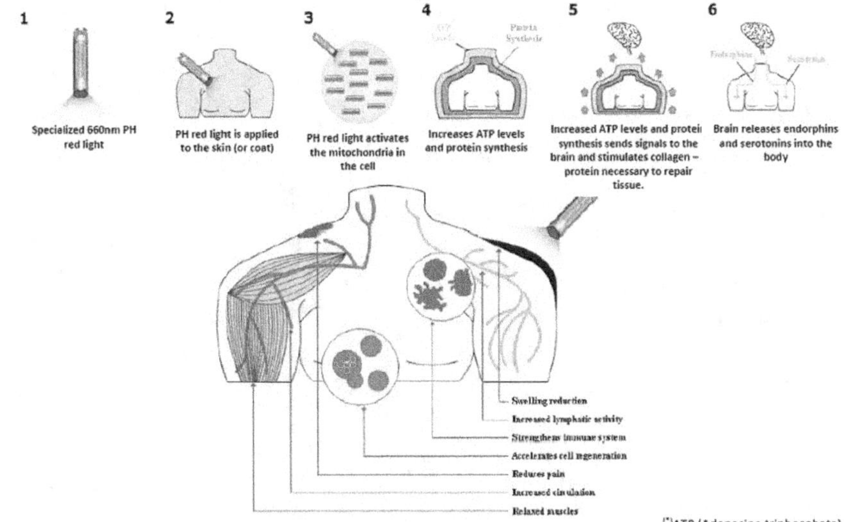

We found and bought our own system in 2015, and have been using it ever since. I've had a few clients along the way, and with that, have collected several testimonies. It has helped me through my chemo treatments, this anti-hormone therapy, and through my reconstruction surgeries as well.

Check out Appendix A for NASA's non-invasive LED-Photodynamic therapy for cancer and wound healing. An abstract that discusses the clinical trials NASA conducted using human subjects.

Weight Loss

How many of you have heard this one… *The best remedies for weight gain are watching your diet and increasing your physical activity.* Basically, calories in… calories out. Okay. And this one… *If you would like more information about how to maintain proper eating habits, you may wish to seek the advice of a registered dietician.* DID THAT TOO!! Do you know what I got?? A prescription for ENSURE! Lovely.

I just recently talked to my oncologist about my anti-hormone prescription and the weight gain it's causing. He said, "Exercise? I'm sorry, but there's no magic pill for that." Sorry? Meanwhile, the extra weight causes other health problems. Needless to say, I've tried a lot of different things to take off the weight. I'm going to share them with you here. Unfortunately for me, I like all kinds of food and I like to try new foods. I don't particularly like fat-free anything or sugar-free anything. I don't feel I'm picky, I just like the full flavor of food. Does that mean I don't eat healthy? Not necessarily. I can eat healthy when I put my mind to it. I also have a great respect for the food choices and lifestyles other people adhere to. I just don't like the word "diet". It turns me off, makes me feel restricted or deprived in choices, and then eating becomes a chore. Eating should never become a chore and it should always be guiltless. It should be enjoyable. "Diets" are temporary. "Lifestyles" are forever. With that being said, let's explore a few food lifestyles.

Mediterranean

This is my favorite food lifestyle. This way of eating was never intended to be used to lose weight. It's a heart healthy lifestyle born in the region around the Mediterranean Sea; Italy, Greece, and Croatia.

This food lifestyle is loaded with fruits and vegetables, whole grains, potatoes, fish, seafood, nuts, legumes and olive oil. Eat poultry, eggs, cheese and yogurt in moderation (how do you eat Italian with moderate cheese?) Rarely eat red meat. It's recommended to avoid sugary drinks, added sugars, processed meat, refined grains, refined oils and other highly processed foods. Meat, fish or poultry should be a side dish with the biggest portion of the meal being vegetables. Plus, you're allowed one 5 oz. glass of red wine per day (men are allowed two glasses). How could you *not* like this way of eating?? The key is eating in moderation.

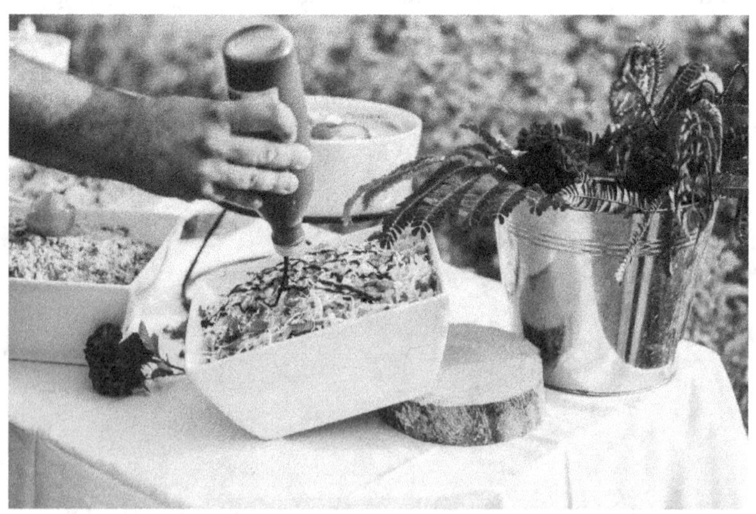

Whole Food Plant Based

I enjoy this food lifestyle as well, but I find it a bit more difficult to jump into. This one needs to be a gradual transition with lots of patience with yourself. The benefits of this healthy lifestyle seem endless. It can lower the risk of prostate, breast and other cancers, prevent and even reverse heart disease, prevent and treat diabetes, helps with weight loss, and increases energy. And the best part… you can eat whenever you're hungry and eat until you're full! There's no starving yourself, fasting, or intermittent fasting (unless you just want to).

Eat these in Abundance

- *Whole grains*: barley, brown rice, teff, millet, wild rice, quinoa, amaranth, steel cut and rolled oats, whole wheat
- *Legumes*(dried or canned with minimal salt): adzuki, beans, black beans, black-eyed-peas, chickpeas, fava beans, kidney beans, soybeans, green beans, peas, mung beans, lentils, lima beans, pinto beans, homemade veggie burgers
- *Greens* (fresh or frozen): kale, collards, spinach, lettuces, parsley, cilantro, chards, bok choy, arugula
- *Roots*: all potatoes, onions, leeks, carrots, radishes, beets, garlic, ginger, turnips, daikon

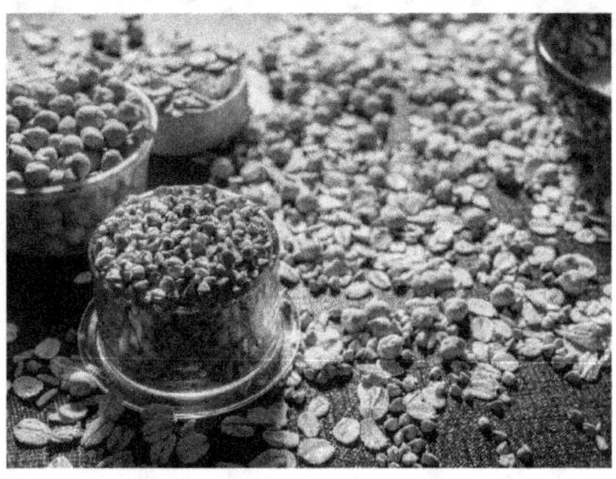

- *Other Veggies*: squash, celery, Brussel sprouts, cauliflower, mushrooms, asparagus, peppers, tomatoes, zucchini, sea vegetables
- *Fruit* (fresh or frozen): apricots, apples, bananas, berries, cherries, melons, mangoes, papayas, pineapple, grapes, kiwi, plums
- *Omega 3 rich seeds*: flaxseed, chia seed
- *Spices*: All spices
- *Beverages*: water, unsweetened plant "milks", herbal teas, decaffeinated coffee

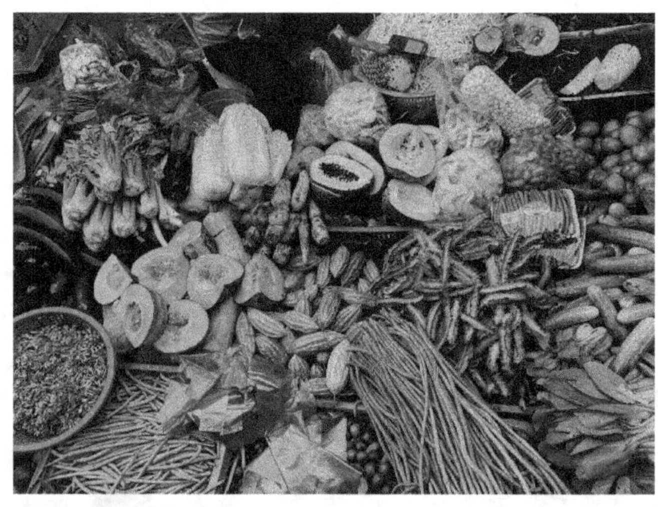

These are considered healthy food, but they are higher in fat and sugar content. So, it's advised to use them sparingly.

- *Nuts*
- *Coconut*
- *Avocado*
- *Seeds*: sesame, pumpkin, sunflower
- *Dried fruit*
- *Added sweeteners*: maple syrup, date syrup, molasses
- *Minimally processed whole soy products*: tofu, tempeh, miso
- *Beverages*: caffeinated coffee and tea, alcohol

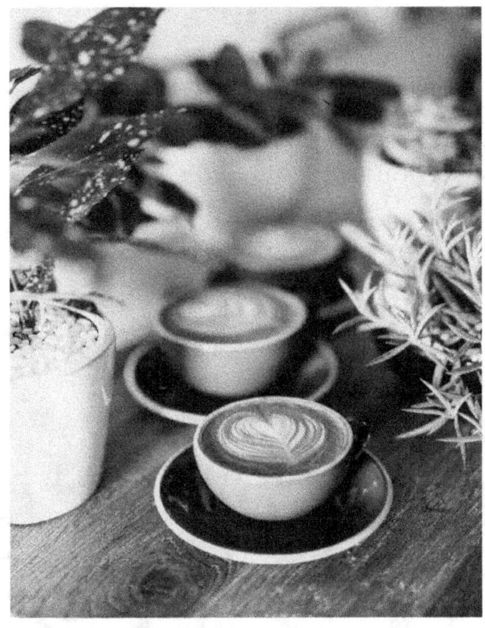

- *Meat*: fish, poultry, seafood, red meat, processed meat
- *Dairy*: yogurt, milk, cheese, butter, half and half, buttermilk
- *Eggs*: chicken, duck, quail, and ostrich?
- *Plant fragments* (these include vegan replacement foods):
- *Added fats*: oils, margarine
- *Refined sugar*: white sugar, barley malt, beet sugar, brown rice syrup, brown sugar, cane juice crystals, cane sugar, corn syrup, confectioner's sugar, fructose
- *Refined grains*: white flour, white rice, quick cook oats
- *Protein Isolates*: soy protein isolate, pea protein isolate, seitan
- *Beverages*: soda, fruit juice (even 100% pure), sports drinks, energy drinks

(nutrition studies – whole food)

Now you can see why the transition needs to be gradual with a lot of patience! Meal planning and prepping for the week or the month usually helps me stay on track.

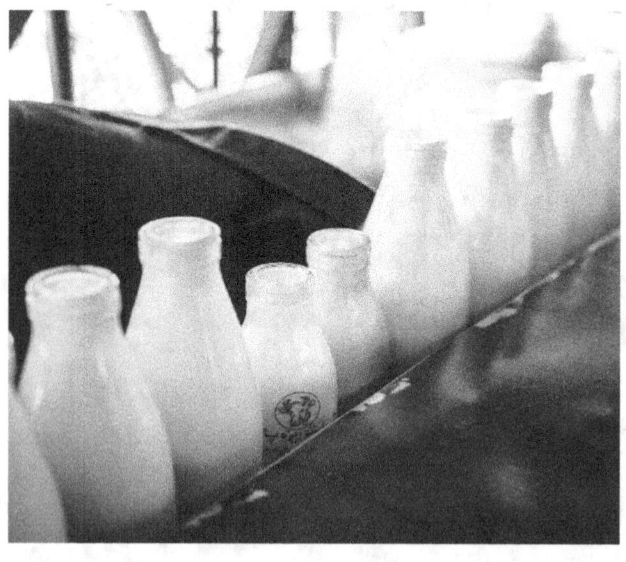

Vegetarian vs. Vegan

A vegetarian is someone who doesn't eat any meat, fish, seafood, poultry, game, or any by-products of animal slaughter (hotdogs, bologna, sausage). There are several types of vegetarians:
- Lacto-ovo vegetarians: avoid all animal flesh, but consume dairy and egg products
- Lacto vegetarians: avoid animal flesh and eggs, but consume dairy products
- Ovo vegetarians: avoid all animal products except eggs
- Vegan: avoid all animal and animal-derived products
- Pescatarians: do not eat meat or poultry, but do eat fish

(Vegan – vegsoc.org)

Vegans have the strictest form of vegetarianism. According to the Vegan Society, veganism is a way of living which seeks to exclude, as far as possible and practicable, all forms of exploitation of, and cruelty to, animals for food, clothing, health, and environment. Vegetarian and Vegan food lifestyles are low in saturated fat and cholesterol, but contain high amounts of vitamins, minerals, and fiber. Poorly planned meals for both lifestyles can result in low intakes of nutrients like iron, calcium, zinc, vitamin D, B12, and the Omega-3s.

I can do the Pescatarian lifestyle. I'm not very good at being a vegetarian (I've tried), although I think I could do it with the right meal planning. Or... maybe not... I fold with outside influence every single time. No will power. <heavy sigh> Does liking the idea count?

Keto

"The keto diet is a very low-car, higher-fat diet. It's similar in many ways to other low-carb diets (Atkins). While you eat far fewer carbohydrates on a keto diet, you maintain moderate protein consumption and may increase your intake of fat. The reduction in carb intake puts your body in a metabolic state called ketosis, where fat, from your diet and from your body, is burned for energy."
(Keto – diet doctor)

Studies have found that this lifestyle is beneficial to a wide variety of different health conditions:
- Heart disease
- Cancer
- Alzheimer's disease
- Epilepsy
- Parkinson's disease
- Polycystic ovary syndrome
- Brain injuries
- Acne

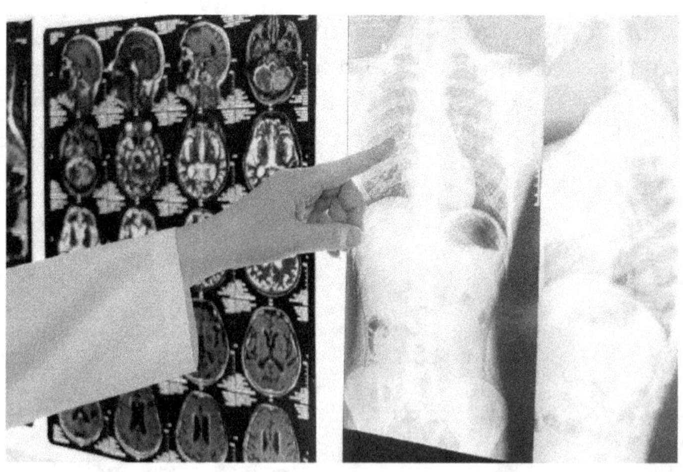

Keto friendly foods:
- Seafood
- Low-Carb Vegetables
- Cheese
- Avocados
- Meat and Poultry
- Eggs
- Coconut Oil
- Plain Greek Yogurt/Cottage Cheese
- Olive Oil
- Nuts and Seeds
- Berries: Blackberries, Blueberries, Raspberries, Strawberries
- Butter and cream
- Shirataki Noodles
- Olives
- Unsweetened Coffee or Tea
- Dark Chocolate/Cocoa Powder

(Keto – Healthline diet foods)

I did this lifestyle while I was going through chemotherapy. Not really the best time to try something new. I eventually gave up and grabbed a twelve pack of tacos on the way home. I haven't tried it since then, but I do have friends that have been very successful with this way of eating. I chose to follow the Diet Doctor and paid a monthly subscription for the extras (meal planning, recipes, etc.). I just wasn't a big fan of counting micronutrients. I still make some of the recipes from this website, since my family also enjoyed them.

Cancer introduced me to juicing. I was told that all the green juice would help fight cancer. So, I bought a juicer, looked up some recipes, and through trial and error even created a few of my own. I'll admit, the first several concoctions were nasty. But, we drank them anyway. Why? Because we thought healthy wasn't supposed to taste good. Boy, was I wrong! My family didn't juice to lose weight, we juiced to get healthy. We usually drank the juice with a meal, or made smoothies with it. It was never a meal substitute, but it did make it easier to meet the daily servings of fruits and vegetables.

I believe that the more rapidly you lose weight, the more rapidly you'll gain it back. When I hear people talking about juicing to lose weight, I think of fasting. You might get the nutrients faster, but you leave out the fiber and protein that your body also needs. People also use juicing to "detox" the body. The liver and kidneys get rid of toxins for you, so I think detoxing isn't really necessary. The key is to be smart about it and listen to what your body needs. And don't juice the orange peel!

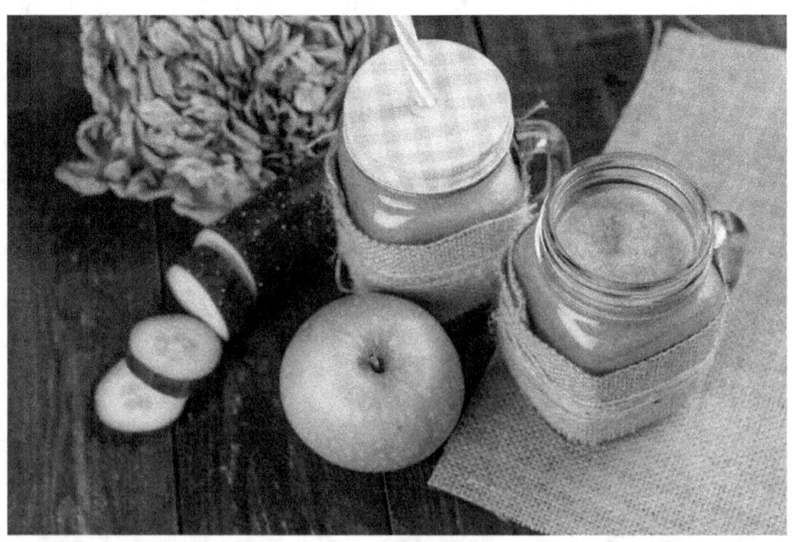

I've never tried this, but I'm curious. It looks like the complete opposite of veganism and seems like it could be unhealthy in the long term.
"The Carnivore Diet is a restrictive diet that only includes meat, fish, and animal foods like eggs and certain dairy products. It excludes all other foods, including fruits, vegetables, legumes, grains, nuts, and seeds." (Carnivore – Healthline)

The controversial belief is that human ancestral populations ate mostly meat and fish and high-carb diets are to blame for today's high rates of chronic disease. It's believed that it can treat depression, anxiety, arthritis, obesity, and diabetes.

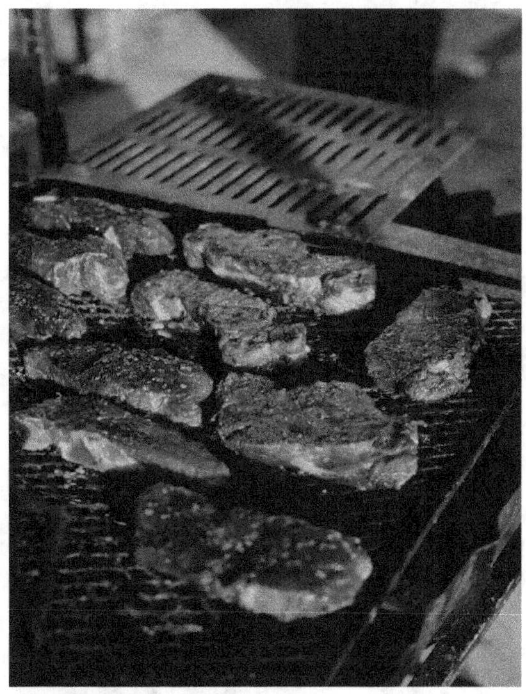

Following this lifestyle is actually very easy. Just eliminate all plant foods from your diet, and eat meat, fish, eggs and small amounts of low-lactose dairy products.

Meat: beef, chicken, pork, lamb, turkey, organ meats, salmon, sardines, white fish
Heavy cream, hard cheese
Butter, lard, bone marrow
Beverages: water, bone broth
Coffee, tea, and any drinks made from plants aren't allowed.
There are no guidelines on calorie intake, meal planning, or serving size. This lifestyle could also be high in fat, cholesterol and sodium; which makes me believe there would be long term health issues.

Because this would be considered a high protein, low-carb diet, it should lead to weight loss. Protein increases your metabolism and helps burn more calories. (Carnivore – md)

If you decide to try this lifestyle, I would love to hear how it works for you, and how your body reacts to it.

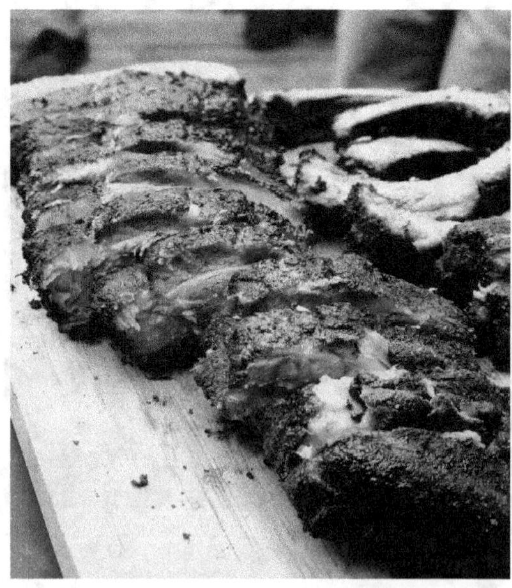

Also called the Paleolithic or caveman diet, this lifestyle is "designed to resemble what human hunter-gatherer ancestors ate thousands of years ago. By following a whole-food based diet and leading physically active lives, hunter-gatherers presumably had much lower rates of lifestyle diseases; obesity, diabetes, heart disease." (Paleo – Healthline)

For the most part, this lifestyle seems super simple. Eat when you're hungry. Eat until you're full, and throw in some exercise for good measure. Here's a rundown of what to eat and what not to eat:

Don't Eat
- Cereal grains
- Legumes (including peanuts)
- Dairy
- Refined sugar, artificial sweeteners, soft drinks, juices
- Potatoes (other websites recommend all Tubers)
- Processed foods, cured meat
- Refined vegetable oils
- Salt (other websites say salt & spices are fine to use)

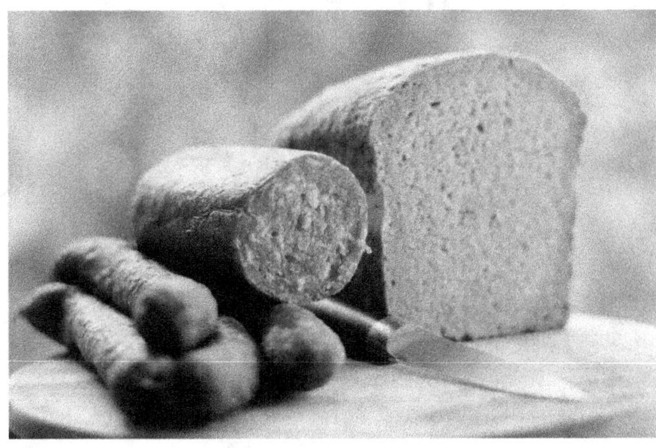

Eat

- Grass produced Meat
- Fish/seafood
- Fresh fruits and veggies
- Eggs
- Nuts and seeds
- Healthful oils (olive, walnut, flaxseed, avocado, coconut)

(Paleo – what to eat)

Again, I have never tried this lifestyle, but I do have a few friends that have given it a try. Most enjoyed it, but felt it was difficult to maintain long term. Some felt it became too expensive, and others thought the lifestyle and food became boring and bland. If you decide to try this lifestyle, I would love to hear about your journey with it.

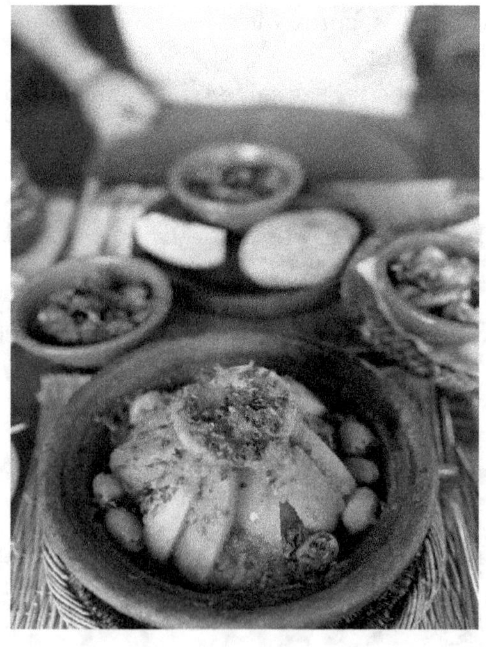

Appetite Suppressants

<u>Legal Disclaimer</u>
In general, the FDA has a limited regulation on OTC or online supplements before they are available for purchase, so use caution when choosing and using supplements. All supplements are not regulated for potency and effectiveness. If you or someone you know is misusing appetite suppressants, it's important to consult your healthcare team.

<u>*Natural Remedy*</u>

For Sugar Cravings:
Gymnema Sylvestre
This amazing herb has been in Ayurvedic medicine for centuries. "The Hindi term for G. Sylvestre is *gurmar*, which translates as 'sugar destroyer'. The leaves contain gymnemic acids, major bioactive ingredients, which suppress the taste of sugar."
(Gymnema – verywellhealth)

According to drug.com, "the plant has been used in traditional medicine, to control blood sugar, as a lipid-lowering agent, for weight loss, and to prevent cavities. As of now, there are no contraindications or interactions with other medications or prescriptions."
(Gymnema – drugs.com)

This stuff actually works for me. I take about ½ tsp. in a cup of water (there's no taste) about 15 to 30 minutes before eating. It definitely makes sweet foods unpleasant. Let's take a look at some additional benefits according to Healthline.

Health Benefits of Gymnema Sylvestre

- Reduces sugar cravings by making sweet foods taste less appealing
- Helps lower blood sugar levels
- May contribute to favorable insulin levels by increasing insulin production
- Improves cholesterol and triglyceride levels, reducing heart disease risk
- May aid in weight loss
- Helps reduce inflammation due to its Tannin and Saponin content

(Gymnema – Healthline)

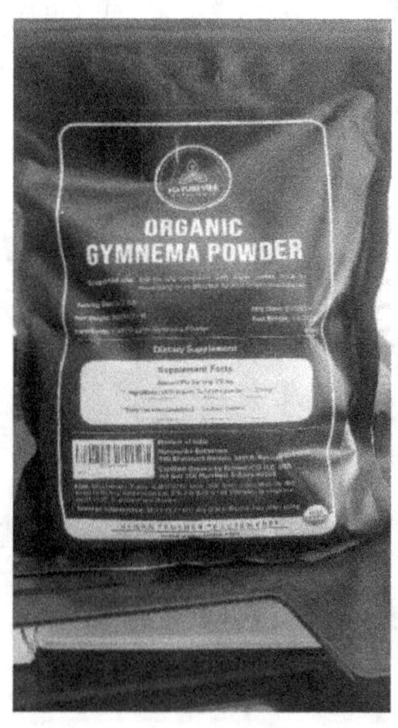

Also known as Konjac Root, this herb grows in different parts of Asia. It's used as a gelatin substitute, and to thicken or add texture to foods or sauces. I've used it in gravy and different sauces to help thicken it. It is well known in traditional Chinese medicine, and used here as a weight loss supplement and for cholesterol management. I usually mix ½ tsp to 1tsp. of the powder with an 8oz. glass of water, 15 to 30 minutes before eating a meal. There is no taste, so you can mix it with anything. I like to mix this with the **Gymnema Powder** in water. I also drink the entire concoction right then. If you wait too long, it gels up and can cause you to choke or gag on it. The pills are not recommended due to the choking hazard. Just be aware!

Konjac Root Glucomannan

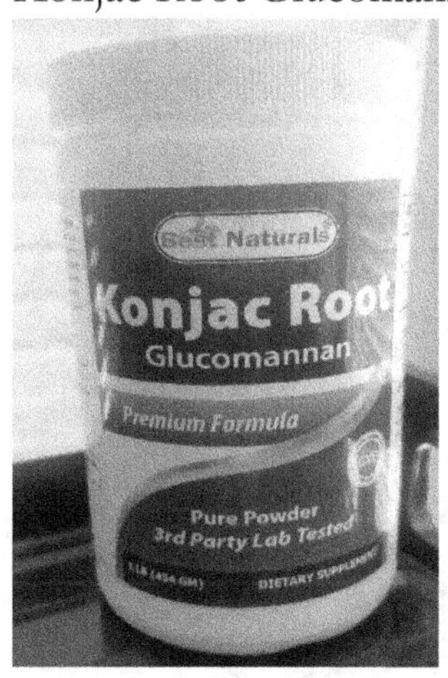

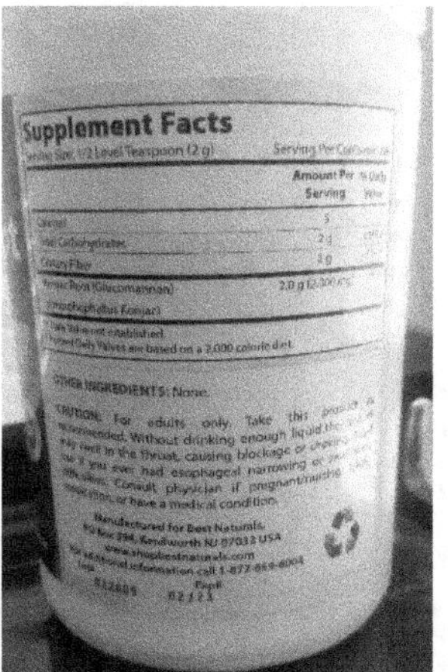

Benefits of Glucomannan

- Weight loss
- Diabetes management
- Reduction in cholesterol levels, LDL (bad cholesterol)
- Prevents constipation
- Improves overall skin health
- Quick wound healing

Higher risk if you:
- Take konjac tablets
- Take konjac in any form without water
- Are elderly
- Have problems swallowing

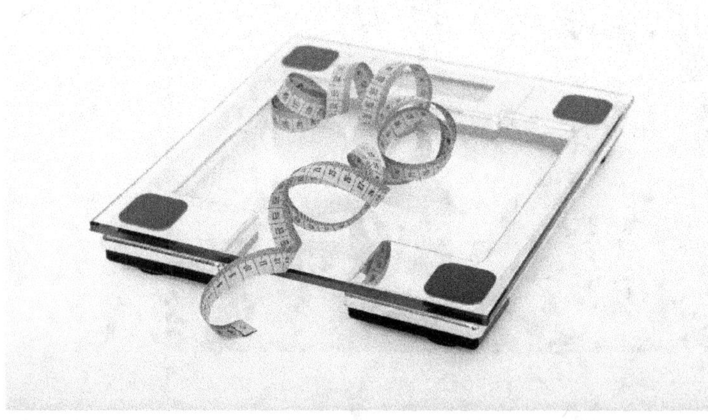

Lipoic Acid

"Lipoic acid is an antioxidant that is found in some foods and is also manufactured in the body. Its primary role seems to be regulating blood sugar, but lipoic acid may also be beneficial in dealing with diabetes, the brain, the liver, blood pressure, glaucoma, cancer cells, scars, and aging in general. It also increases the effectiveness of other antioxidants, like vitamins." (Lipoic Acid – prime women)

It sounds like a wonder drug, doesn't it?

"As of August 2020, this supplement has been undergoing clinical trials in Asia, Europe, New Zealand and the United States. Out of 13 clinical trials, 10 have reported weight loss or a decrease in BMI. Another issue is the formulation of the supplement. Many previous studies have used the S-form of lipoic acid, which is a product of industrial synthesis and not found in nature." In the clinical trials conducted in the United States, "only the R-form of lipoic acid - the form found in the body naturally."
(Lipoic Acid – nutraingredients)

Alli

"Alli is the over-the-counter version of a pharmaceutical weight loss drug called Orlistat. The prescription only version is called Xenical, which contains a higher dosage. Alli contains 60mg of orlistat, while Xenical contains 120mg. It's usually prescribed for long-term obesity management, alongside a low-fat, calorie-restricted diet."
(Alli – Healthline)

"This pill is a lipase inhibitor. It works by reducing the absorption of fat in your body. You take the pill three times per day (one hour before, during, or after each meal). Some side effects include: gas, loose or oily stools, stomach cramps, oily spotting on your underwear, and difficulty controlling bowel movements." (Alli – verywellfit)

Other benefits include reduction in type 2 diabetes, blood pressure, and of total- and LDL cholesterol. There's also a possibility that it could interfere with the absorption of some medications. Is it worth it? With the type of medications we're taking, I wouldn't recommend it, but definitely talk to your doctor before trying it out.

Leanbean

I've never tried this supplement, but it had high reviews. I'd thought I'd research them and provide you another option. The main ingredient in this supplement is glucomannan. If you remember in our previous discussion the risk in taking glucomannan in pill form. This pill has 3000mg of Konjac Root, but has also added several other vitamins and minerals for overall health and wellness.

Added ingredients:
- Choline
- Vitamin B6, B12
- Chromium Picolinate
- Chloride
- Zinc
- Green Coffee
- Turmeric
- Garcinia Cambogia
- Acai Berry
- Piperine

Zotrim

An herbal weight loss aid that claims to reduce feelings of hunger within a few days. There are clinical trials and published studies that support this supplement. You can find the links in the Resources section. The patent comes from the European Patent Office, and there are more published articles in scientific journals than clinical trial reports. It looks like this product comes from the UK. If you decide to give it a try, tell me about your overall experience.

Ingredients:
- Yerba Mate-Leaf Extract
- Guarana-Seed Extract
- Damiana-Leaf Extract
- Caffeine
- Vitamin B3, B6

Pure Garcinia Cambogia
Garcinia Cambogia is a small, pumpkin shaped, yellow or greenish fruit. Supplements are made from the extracts of the fruit's peel. The active substance is hydroxycitric acid (HCA).

Benefits:
- Reduce appetite
- Block fat production, reduce belly fat
- Decreases insulin levels
- Decreases leptin levels
- Reduces inflammation
- Improves blood sugar
- Increases insulin sensitivity

(Garcinia – Healthline)

There have been a few reports of side effects when using this product; digestive issues, headaches or skin rashes. A more serious side effect is liver damage or liver failure. I've included a clinical study/case study for your review: (Garcinia – ncbi.nlm.nih.gov)

I've taken this supplement in the past without any change in weight. I could say it was the product, but it could have easily been my eating habits, or a lack of exercise. Anyway, I do believe if you're going to take a supplement then it needs to be paired with a healthy food lifestyle and a good exercise plan for the best results. I'm not always very good at staying consistent with any plan. I start out with a bang, then fizzle out like a wet firecracker.

Phentermine Hydrochloride (Adipex-P, Lomaira, Suprenza)

One of the most popular weight loss drugs in the world, phentermine hydrochloride has been proven effective for short-term weight loss when used in conjunction with a healthy food lifestyle and exercise.

"Because of its chemical similarities to amphetamine, it's considered a controlled substance and can only be prescribed by a doctor. The drug supposedly increases the chemical messengers, norepinephrine, serotonin, and dopamine in the brain. When the levels of these three chemicals increase, the feeling of hunger decreases." (Phentermine – Healthline)

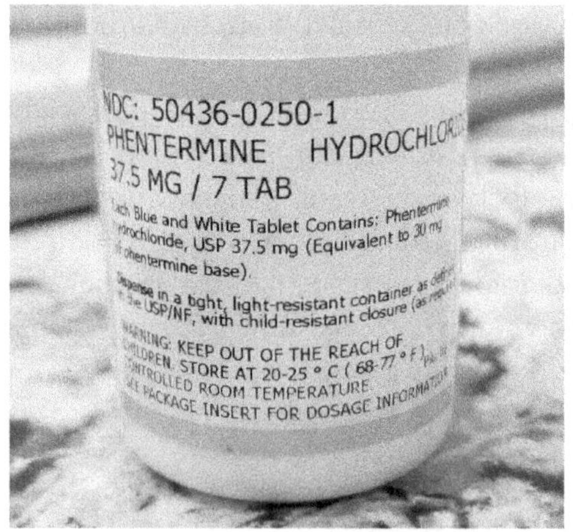

Of course, every medication has *side effects*:
-    Dry mouth
-    Sleeping problems
-    Dizziness
-    Heart palpitations
-    Flushing of the skin
-    Fatigue
-    Constipation
-    Irritability

Don't take this medication if you have:
-    A history of heart disease
-    Severe or uncontrolled high blood pressure
-    Overactive thyroid
-    Glaucoma
-    Extreme agitation or nervousness
-    A history of drug abuse
-    If you're taking other diet pills
-    Used an MAO inhibitor within the last 14 days

(Phentermine – drugs.com)

Qsymia

"This drug contains a combination of phentermine and topiramate in an extended-release capsule. Phentermin is an appetite suppressant, and Topiramate is used as a seizure medication. Together with the proper diet and exercise it's used to treat obesity. It's also used to treat obesity that's related to diabetes, high cholesterol or high blood pressure.
It's important to tell your doctor if you have high blood pressure, heart disease, diabetes, liver or kidney disease, low blood levels of potassium or have had a heart attack or stroke within the past six months."
(Qsymia – drugs.com)

Orlistat

I discussed this medication in the "over-the-counter appetite suppressant" section. "The prescription name for this drug is Xenical. It blocks some of the fat that you eat, and keeps it from being absorbed by your body. It can be used for weight loss or to help reduce the risk of regaining weight already lost. As always, it must be used with a healthy food lifestyle and exercise. It's only for adults that are overweight or obese."
(Orlistat – drugs.com)

Exercise, Workout Plans, & Equipment

Since I've retired in 2015, I haven't been the greatest at maintaining a good exercise regimen. It's really not my favorite thing to do; although I know it's good for me. Since my cancer diagnosis, I also know exercise is important to ensure that there's no future recurrence. But, unfortunately, it's still a struggle for me. My cancer journey added about 30lbs, and the anti-hormone therapy has added another 20lbs. In September 2020, I weighed in at 206 lbs. I was mesmerized, and now wished I had taken a picture of the scale reading because I still can't believe it. I'm still absolutely amazed at what these drugs, medications, or chemo do to our bodies! I've started some working out, but nothing 100% serious or consistent. I do swim laps in the pool, and use a kickboard to specifically work out the hips, butt and thighs. I also have a treadmill that I use to walk, and on occasion, a slow jog. I'm still in the worst shape that I've ever been in my life.

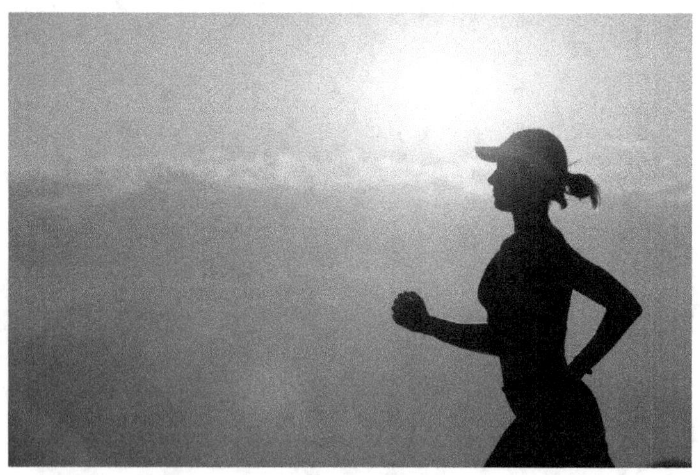

Today, I did 20 attempts to do one sit-up; so I'll just call those crunches... my abs are sore! I do wall push-ups too; my triceps are feeling those! Yes, I joke about this, but I tell you this because we all have to start somewhere. I know that I can't run 2-4 miles anymore or do pushups and sit-ups like I did in the military, but I *do* have to start somewhere, and start safely. The following exercises, workout plans and equipment are just a guideline. Do what's best for your body. Do what's safe for you. But *do* something. I'll be doing it too!

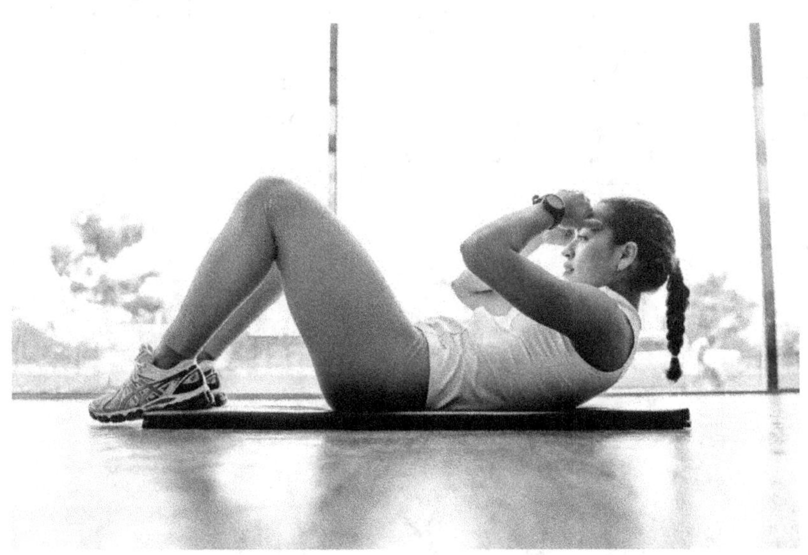

Like I said before, we all know the importance of exercise. We understand the need for a regular exercise routine for our physical health, our mental health, and our emotional health. When I was younger, I was pretty good at staying in shape. It still wasn't my favorite thing to do, but I knew what I had to do and most of the time maintained that. After chemo threw me into menopause, I found that the exercise routine I had used for so long, no longer worked. My body had changed, but I soon found out that the "rules" of exercise had also changed. For example, it's always been told that a good exercise routine should be 30-60 minutes per day, or more if you have the time. Now, as long as you do 15 minutes of a high-intensity activity that gets your heart pumping and leaves you breathless, you're good! It can "kick start your metabolic rate, reduce body fat, and increase muscle mass."

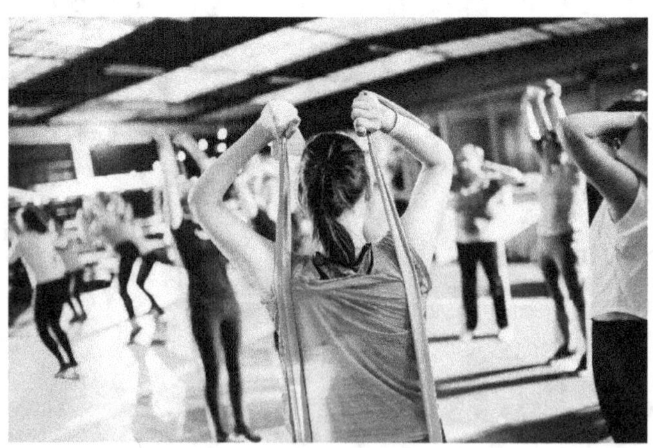

Let's take a look at some other benefits of exercise:

- Boosts brain power: regular exercise may play an important role in protecting your brain from Alzheimer's disease
- Prevents osteoporosis: aerobic exercise, resistance training, and Tai Chi improves balance and muscle strength
- Helps our muscles age well
- Better sex
- Better sleep
- Better digestion
- Helps manage stress, lowers risk of anxiety or depression
- Reduces the risk of cancer: colon, breast
- Decreases stroke risk
- Improves skin

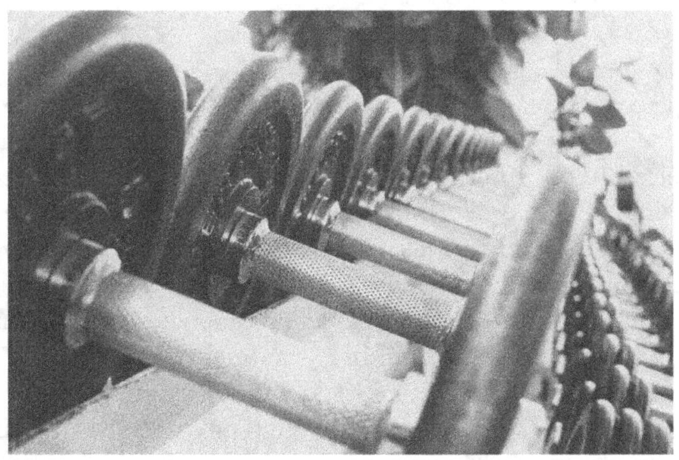

Less is more. "Science currently suggests that for all populations' high intensity and low intensity workouts reap more optimal results. If you're in menopause, there is more proof. First, moderate exercise has little to no association with improvements in helping hot flashes. Second, the higher the fitness level upon entering menopause the reduced menopause symptoms women report. Higher levels of fitness occur from exercise of adequate intensity. High-intensity interval training and strength training performed to the point of muscular fatigue are two ways to reach adequate intensity. Moderate intensity level exercise falls into the 'no benefits zone'." (Exercise – Prime Women moderate)

Four types of exercise

It's important to get all four types of exercise into your routine because each one has a different benefit. One can help improve the others, and some exercises have all four in one. Again, it's what works best for you and your body.

Endurance
Anything that increases your heart rate or breathing is considered an endurance activity or an aerobic exercise. Increasing your endurance levels releases endorphins; which, results in a positive mind set. The act of gaining endurance through physical activity decreases anxiety, depression, stress and various chronic diseases. As I said before, less is more. High intensity interval training (HIIT), quick sessions of intense exercise, improves endurance in conjunction with traditional training. For example, when running the track, sprint the straightaways and jog the curves. Add some strength. Variation is important. Resistance training can strengthen our bones, ligaments, tendons, and muscles. Mixing up aerobic exercise with kettlebells, dumbbells, and body weight exercises improves stamina and overall endurance. People will often find their fitness niche and stick only to that regime. It's important to incorporate a variety of exercises in order to build endurance. If it's not a challenge, then the workout isn't beneficial.

Train smart.
Training smart means training safely. To avoid injury, increase the fitness routine gradually, drink plenty of water, get plenty of rest, and allow the body to heal.

Endurance exercises
- Walking or jogging
- Dancing
- Swimming
- Biking
- Climbing stairs
- Hiking
- Playing tennis or basketball

*Tip: If you're breathing hard but can still have a conversation easily, it's moderate-intensity. If you can only say a few words before you have to take a breath, it's high-intensity.

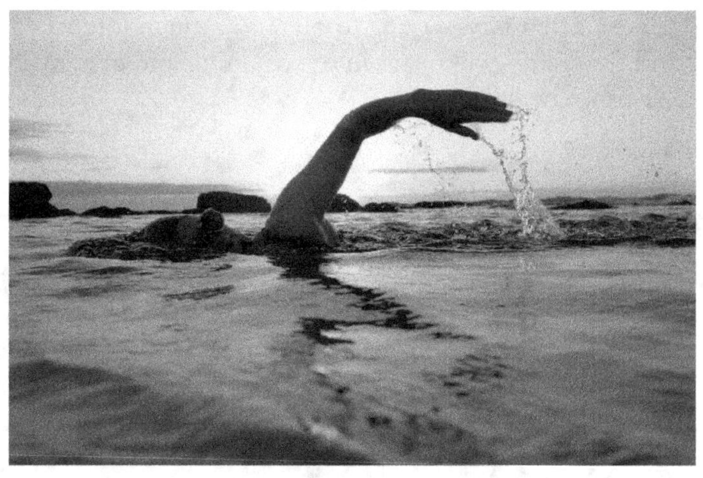

Strength training specializes in the use of resistance to induce muscular contraction; which builds anaerobic endurance, and the size of skeletal muscles. When properly performed, strength training can provide significant functional benefits and improvement in overall health and well-being. These include: weight loss, increased bone, muscle, tendon and ligament strength and toughness; improved joint function, reduced potential for injury, increased bone density, increased metabolism, improved cardiac function and elevated HDL (good) cholesterol. It's also important to use a variety of exercises and types of equipment to target specific muscle groups.

There are three important variables of strength training; intensity, volume, and frequency. Intensity refers to the amount of work required to achieve the activity, and is proportional to the mass of the weights being lifted. Volume refers to the number of muscles worked, exercises, sets and repetitions during a single session. Frequency refers to how many training sessions are performed per week. Increasing one by any significant amount necessitates the decrease of the other two. Trying to push too much intensity, volume and frequency will result in overtraining and eventually lead to injury or other health issues.

So with all this information, what exercises do I do?

When it comes to strength training, all muscle groups need to be worked to avoid muscle imbalances. As a beginner, choose one to two exercises for each muscle group in the upper body, and three to four for the lower body.

Muscle groups
- Chest: bench press, chest press machine, pushups
- Back: seated row machine, back extensions, lateral pull-downs
- Shoulders: overhead press, lateral raise, front raise
- Biceps: bicep curls, hammer curls, concentration curls
- Triceps: triceps extensions, dips, kickbacks
- Lower body: squats, lunges, leg press machines, deadlifts, calf raises
- Abdominals: crunches, reverse crunches, oblique twists, pelvic tilts

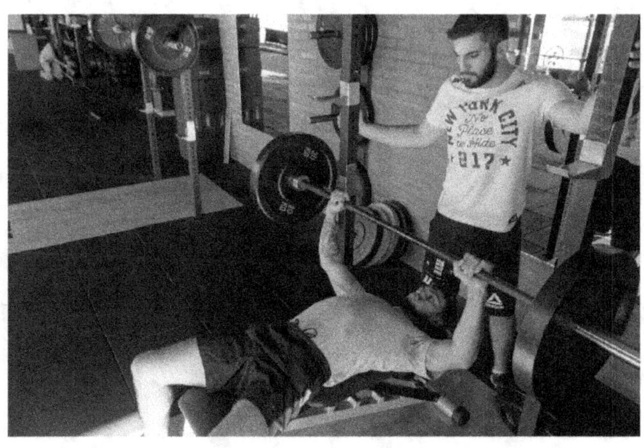

Repetitions, sets and weight can be confusing when conducting strength training. This is determined by personal goal sets. Here's a goal guide:

To lose body fat: Use the amount of weight that allows a completion of *only* ten to twelve repetitions and one to three sets (one set for beginners, two to three sets for intermediate and advanced exercisers). Rest for 30 second to one minute between sets, and at least one day between workout sessions.

For muscle gain: Use the amount of weight that allows a completion of *only* four to eight repetitions and three or more sets. Rest for one to two minutes between sets and two to three days between sessions. We often do one muscle group per day. For beginners, condition for several weeks before weight training with this degree of difficulty. A "spotter" is highly recommended.

For health and endurance: Use the amount of weight that allows a completion of *only* twelve to sixteen repetitions, one to three sets, and a resting period of 20-30 seconds. Allow for a minimum of one day between workout sessions.

To determine how much weight should be used, start with a light weight and perform one set. Add weight until the desired number of repetitions can be accomplished. The last repetitions should be difficult, but not impossible, and maintain good form.

*Tip: Resistance bands are stretchy elastic bands that come in several strengths, from light to heavy. You can use them in some strength exercises instead of weights.

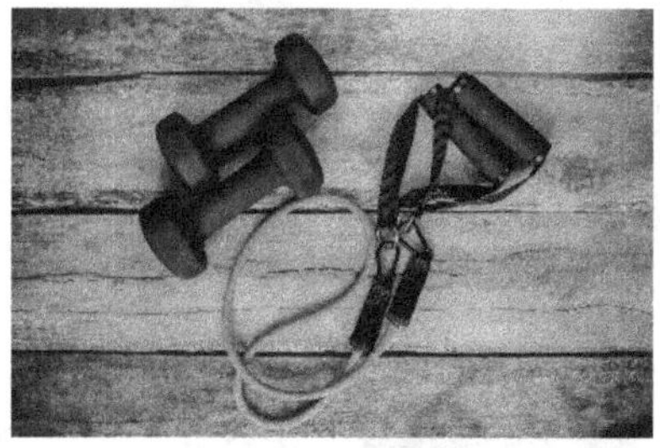

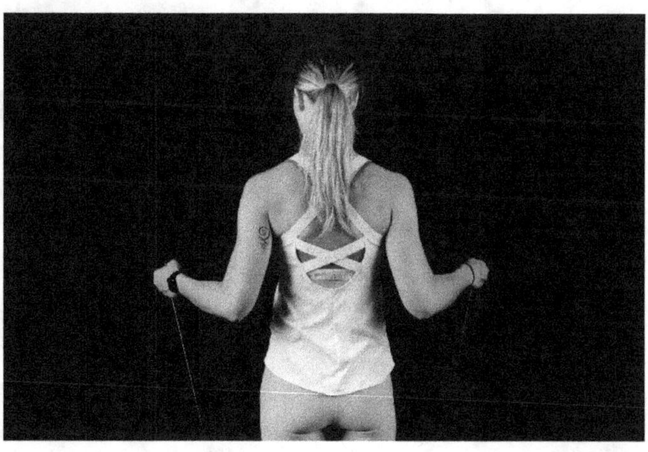

Flexibility or limberness refers to the absolute range of movement in a joint or series of joints, and lengthen muscles that cross the joints to induce a bending movement or motion. This varies between individuals, particularly in terms of differences in muscle length of multi-joint muscles. The flexibility in some joints increases to a certain degree with exercise, but stretching is the common component to maintaining or improving limberness.

The quality of life is enhanced by improving and maintaining a good range of motion in the joints. Overall, flexibility should be developed with a specific joint, range of motion in mind. Many factors are taken into account when establishing personal flexibility: joint structure, ligaments, tendons, muscles, skin, tissue injury, fat (adipose) tissue, body temperature, activity level, age and gender all influence an individual's range of motion surrounding a joint.

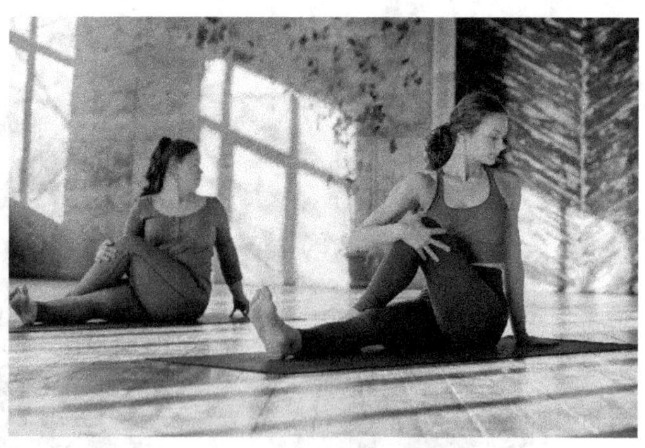

It's important to include flexibility training as part of a regular fitness routine. Improved flexibility enhances performance in aerobic training, and muscular conditioning. The incidence of injury decreases when people include flexibility training in their daily routines. This is due to the ability to move unimpeded through a wider range of motion. When used appropriately, flexibility training allows you to connect with your body. Stretching is a form of active relaxation that improves mental and physical recovery after completing a challenging workout; there is a focus on relaxation and the rejuvenation of the mind and body.

After pushing the body to work hard, it's time to encourage recovery. This is an excellent time for flexibility training because the muscles are warm and pliable, allowing them to stretch farther. The following are some of the major benefits of flexibility training:
Reduces stress in exercising muscles and releases tension developed during the workout.
Assists with posture by balancing the tension placed across the joint by the muscles that cross it. Proper posture minimizes stress and maximizes the strength of all joint movements.
Reduces the risk of injury during exercise and daily activities because muscles are more pliable.
Improves performance of everyday activities as well as performance in exercise and sport.

Choose activities that serve two functions: relaxation and flexibility. There are many methods of flexibility training that promote relaxation:
- Yoga
- Mediation
- Pilates
- Tai Chi
- Breathing exercises

These are natural alternatives to assist you in relaxing; encourage yourself to de-stress from your busy life.

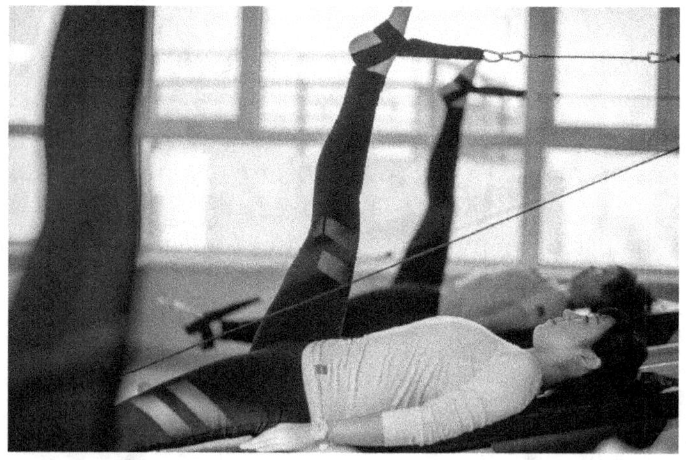

Given that balance performance is affected by muscle strength and flexibility, resistance training and stretching programs may be useful for maintaining and improving balance. In addition to increasing strength and range of motion, Pilates, yoga, tai chi, dance, walking and combinations of exercise modalities are also suitable activities for improving balance. Balance discs, foam pads and rollers, balance boards, stability balls, and computerized balance training systems are tools that add variety and challenge to balance training programs. A strong core is also responsible for your sense of balance.

Maintaining balance is coordinated by three systems. The first is the vestibular or auditory system, located in the inner ear to keep you level. The second balance coordinator is the proprioceptive system, which uses sensory nerves called proprioceptors that are located in the muscles, tendons, and joints. They give signals to the central nervous system, which gives you a kinesthetic sense, or an awareness of your body posture and spatial awareness. Finally, there is the visual system, which sends visual signals from the eyes to the brain about your body's position in relation to its surroundings.

Tai Chi is perfect for balance exercise and core strengthening. Tai Chi is practiced in a variety of styles; Yang and Wu. They have their own movements and traditional length of practice. The Yang style uses a wide stance and steady, slow speed of movement with constant knee flexion. Shifting body weight in this stance demands strength and flexibility. In contrast, the Wu style uses higher stances with a narrower stance width and slower movements, requiring more balance than strength; which may be more appropriate for balance training programs.

Originally developed for self-defense, Tai Chi has evolved into a graceful form of exercise that is now used for stress reduction and for a variety of other health conditions. Often described as meditation in motion, Tai Chi is a noncompetitive, self-paced system of gentle physical exercise and stretching. Each posture flows into the next without pause, ensuring that your body is in constant motion.

When learned correctly and performed regularly, Tai Chi can be a positive part of an overall approach to improving your health.

Benefits
- Decreased stress and anxiety
- Enhance quality of sleep
- Increased aerobic capacity
- Enhance the immune system
- Increased energy and stamina
- Lower cholesterol levels and blood pressure
- Increased flexibility, balance and agility
- Improve joint pain
- Increased muscle strength and definition
- Reduces risk of falls in older adults

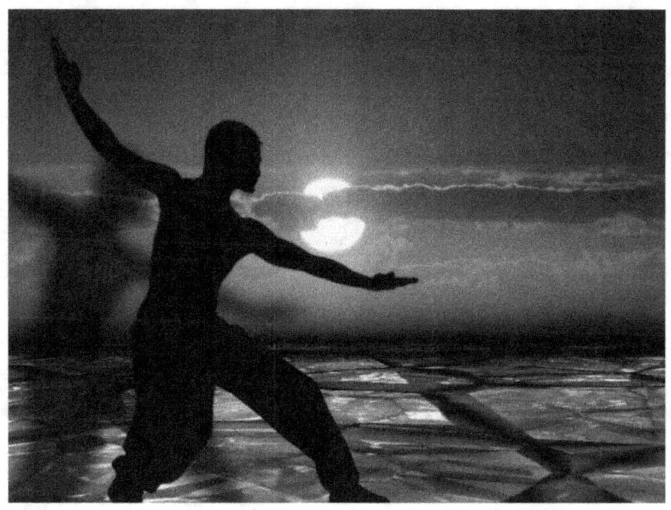

Exercise Plans:

WEIGHT LIFTING/ISO	MONDAY LBS/REP	TUESDAY LBS/REP	WEDNESDAY LBS/REP	THURSDAY LBS/REP	FRIDAY LBS/REP	SATURDAY LBS/REP
CHEST						
BENCH PRESS						
BENCH PRESS ISO						
BENCH PRESS MACHINE						
MACHINE FLYS						
DUMBELL FLYS						
CABLE FLYS						
INCLINES BENCH PRESS						
INCLINES ISO						
INCLINES BENCH MACHINE						
DECLINES BENCH PRESS						
DECLINES ISO						
DECLINES BENCH MACHINE						
PUSHUPS						
TRX PUSHUPS						

WEIGHT LIFTING/ISO	MONDAY LBS/REP	TUESDAY LBS/REP	WEDNESDAY LBS/REP	THURSDAY LBS/REP	FRIDAY LBS/REP	SATURDAY LBS/REP
SHOULDERS						
SHOULDER PRESS ISO						
SHOULDER PRESS MACHINE						
DUMBELL						
SHOULDER FLYS CABLE						
INVERTED CABLE FLYS						
SHOULDER FLYS MACHINE						

WEIGHT LIFTING/ISO	MONDAY LBS/REP	TUESDAY LBS/REP	WEDNESDAY LBS/REP	THURSDAY LBS/REP	FRIDAY LBS/REP	SATURDAY LBS/REP
BACK						
LAT ISO						
FRONT PULLDOWNS WIDE GRIP 90 DEG						
PULLDONW BACK						
FRONT PULLDOWNS MID GRIP 30 DEG						
CABLE BACK						
KETTLE BELLS						
LATES FREEMO						
UNDERGRIP TIGHTGRIP 30 DEG						
SEATED ROW						
DUMBELL PULL UPS						
TRAPS PULLUP CABLE						
TRAPS PULLUP BARBELL						

WEIGHT LIFTING/ISO	MONDAY LBS/REP	TUESDAY LBS/REP	WEDNESDAY LBS/REP	THURSDAY LBS/REP	FRIDAY LBS/REP	SATURDAY LBS/REP
ARMS TRICEPS						
CRAZY CURLS BARBELL						
CABLE EXT PUSHDOWN						
INVERTED EXT CABLE						
ROPE PULLDOWN CABLE						
CABLE FRONT EXTENSION ONE ARM						
TRICEP MACHINE						
DIPS						
TRICEP DUMBELL EXT						
TRICEP BENCH						

WEIGHT LIFTING/ISO	MONDAY LBS/REP	TUESDAY LBS/REP	WEDNESDAY LBS/REP	THURSDAY LBS/REP	FRIDAY LBS/REP	SATURDAY LBS/REP
ARMS BICEPS						
BICEP BARBELL SEATED						
DUMBELLS						
CABLE CURLS						
ROPE CABLE						
BICEP MACHINE						
BICEP PULLUPS						
CABLE BICEPS						
BICEP DOUBLE UP						
SEATED BICEP ISO						

WEIGHT LIFTING/ISO	MONDAY LBS/REP	TUESDAY LBS/REP	WEDNESDAY LBS/REP	THURSDAY LBS/REP	FRIDAY LBS/REP	SATURDAY LBS/REP
LEGS						
LEG EXT						
LEG CURL						
CALF MACHINE						
SQUAT MACHINE						

CARDIO	MONDAY REPS/TIME	TUESDAY REPS/TIME	WEDNESDAY REPS/TIME	THURSDAY REPS/TIME	FRIDAY REPS/TIME	SATURDAY REPS/TIME
ABS						
ELIPTICLE						
RUN						
KNUCKLE PUSHUPS						
FINGER TIP PUSHUPS						
INVERTED PUSHUPS						
TRX PUSHUPS						
TRX PULLUPS						
8 COUNT BODY BUILDERS						

SWIM ROUTINES	MONDAY LAPS/TIME	TUESDAY LAPS/TIME	WEDNESDAY LAPS/TIME	THURSDAY LAPS/TIME	FRIDAY LAPS/TIME	SATURDAY LAPS/TIME
SWIM - FREE STYLE						
SWIM - SIDE STROKE						
SWIM - BACK STROKE						
SWIM - BREAST STROKE						
SWIM - UNDERWATER						
SWIM - COMBAT SWIM						
SWIM - HOLD BREATH						

FLEXIBILITY/BALANCE	MONDAY TIME	TUESDAY TIME	WEDNESDAY TIME	THURSDAY TIME	FRIDAY TIME	SATURDAY TIME
STRETCHING						
YOGA						
TAI CHI						
PILATES						
MEDITATION						
BREATHING						

Through the years, we've all used some kind of workout equipment. We've been in and out of the gym, utilized personal treadmills, bikes, and ellipticals. Some of us have experience with hand weights, machine weights, and kettlebells. I've done Yoga, and Tai Chi. I've even ungracefully tried Zumba and traditional Aerobics. When the COVID-19 Pandemic swarmed around the world, as you know, everything came to a halt; including access to the gym. During this time, my family figured out ways to keep in shape at home. We already have a treadmill, but with our move from Texas to Florida, we inherited a pool as well. So, now we had running, walking, and swimming available. We eventually invested in a couple of resistance bands sets for a full body workout, chin-up/dip bar, and a couple bags of sand to replace the kettlebells. As establishments slowly began to open, we would go hiking or kayaking just to enjoy the fresh air. Now that gyms have reopened, I can't imagine ever going back to one!

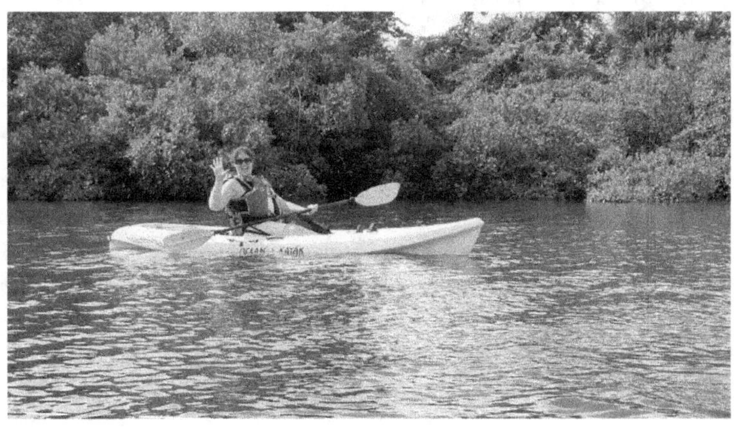

The following lists are only a small example of the equipment that can be utilized to work each specific training segments. Use what's best for you, and within your scope of health and wellness.

Strength training
- Pull-up bar
- Resistance bands sets
- Kettlebells
- Sandbags
- Medicine ball
- Hand weights
- Incline bench
- Suspension straps (TRX training)
- Battle ropes

Cardio training
- Treadmill
- Stationary bike
- Stair climber (unless you have stairs in your house)
- Elliptical (easier on the knees than the treadmill)
- Rowing machine (my favorite)
- Weighted medicine ball

Yoga
- Mat
- Block
- Bag
- Sliders (circular discs)
- Foam roller (don't use on the lower back area)

Outdoors
- Camelback/water
- Backpack
- Mountain bike
- Kayak/Canoe

Cancer Trauma & PTSD

I know I've discussed brain health, chemo brain, brain fog and a few supplements that may help with focus and memory. But, I also feel that mental health as a whole is also very important. Especially in the scope of trauma. Cancer trauma. The entire process is traumatic.

When you hear, "I'm sorry. You have cancer." Fear creeps into your mind. It causes an emotional reaction; sorrow, panic, anxiety. It may cause a physical response; tears, nausea, fatigue. An everlasting effect of trauma sets in. With each new stage or process of the cancer journey (biopsy, chemotherapy, mastectomy or lumpectomy, radiation and every test in between), there comes a new fear of the unknown. And with each new fear, additional emotions attach themselves; adding to the ever-growing trauma. Now, when we add the physical side effects of each medical treatment and the emotional toll that accompanies it, the trauma continues to grow. For example, when we start chemotherapy, the multiple emotions that course through our minds can be debilitating all by itself. After that session, we go home. We sleep. We may be sick. Food may not have any taste. We start to lose our hair. The stress, anxiety, fear, and sorrow permeates. There is continual fear of the unknown. The biggest one being, "Will I live to see tomorrow."

When the last chemo treatment has taken place and we ring the bell of victory, there's a sense of accomplishment, and a heavy weight has been lifted. As the official words of "remission" travel through the air, we breathe a sigh of relief and celebrate. Despite all this, there's still a nagging doubt in the back of our mind. What if my cancer comes back? Can I keep it from coming back? Do I have to take this medication? Is there an alternative or holistic approach in prevention? These nagging thoughts never leave us. They always linger somewhere in the recesses of our minds.

Because these experiences, emotions, and nagging thoughts have become imprinted in the brain, the possibility of being triggered emotionally is very likely. Triggers can be a color, sound, smell or movement that causes a sudden panic, anxiety, or fear. The intensity can range from extremely high to very low. This a form of post-traumatic stress disorder.

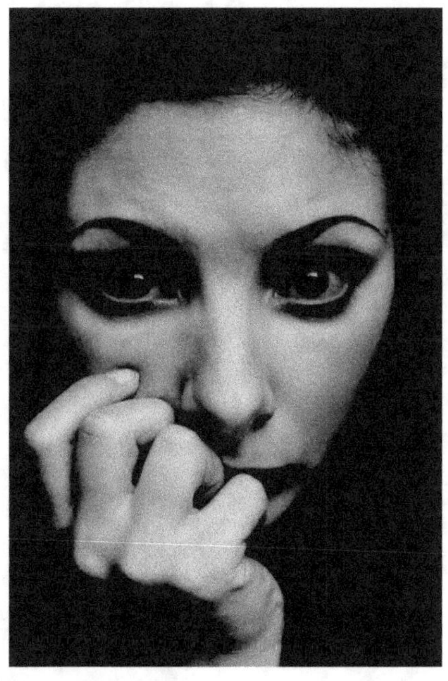

According to breastcancer.org, "about 80% of women have post-traumatic stress disorder (PTSD) symptoms after breast cancer diagnosis." These symptoms don't always appear immediately, but will likely appear within the first three months. There are occasions where symptoms won't develop for at least three to five years. Here are a few symptoms to be aware of:

- Sadness/depression
- Bouts of crying/weepiness
- Memory/concentration problems
- Trouble sleeping
- Shame/guilt
- Hopelessness/helplessness

To manage PTSD symptoms and prevent them from getting worse, it's important to schedule an appointment with your provider as soon as possible. Ask family or friends for help if it get overwhelming or overbearing. Call 911 if you feel suicidal or feel like harming someone else. Forms of treatment may include anti-depressants and/or therapy.

*Look for a book on this in the near future; hopefully, within the next year!

Project Rebuild

The saying goes, "All good things must come to an end." As women, we *are* good things. *And* as women, there should never be an "end". We are never-ending projects and we are always rebuilding ourselves. Rebuilding physically, emotionally, mentally, and spiritually. But most importantly, beautifully. I love that about us. I love that we are all so diverse in culture, race, religion, likes and dislikes. What is even more amazing is how we come together under the wonderful umbrella of womanhood. The horrors of breast cancer unite us even tighter. We embrace each other, support each other, love, laugh and cry for each other.

My hope is that this book has helped connect the dots in the medical unknown. I'm sure some of it was repetitive of what you've already heard and learned from your provider. But, I also hope that there was information that you could take with you. Maybe there was something within these pages that sparked an idea for a wholesome solution for your particular situation, your body and your soul. Whatever it may be, I hope you found it here.

Through the writing of each word, I felt a sense of connection with all of you. Sister to sister. Woman to woman.
And now, I'm finding it hard to finish these last words. I hope to meet you someday. Meet me in social media. Meet in person. Let's connect. Let's *rebuild* our *projects* together.

www.facebook.com/groups/projectrebuild/

Appendix A

The NASA Light-Emitting Diode Medical Program - Progress in Space Flight and Terrestrial Applications

Harry T. Whelan, M.D.[1,2,3,] John M. Houle, B.S.[1]

Noel T. Whelan, I[3] Deborah L. Donohoe, .S., L.A.T.G.[1]

Joan Cwiklinski, M.S.N., C.P.N.P.[1] Meic H. Schmidt, M.DY, Lisa Gould, M.D., Ph.D. lb , David L. Larson, M.D.[1]

Glenn A. Meyer, **M.D** .[1] Vita Cevenini3, Helen Stinson, **B.S.**[3]

I a Departments of Neurology, I b Plastic Surgery and I c Neurosurgery, Medical College of Wisconsin, Milwaukee, WI 53226, (414) 456-4090 [2]Naval Special Warfare Group TWO, Norfolk, VA 23521, (757) 462-7759 3NASA-Marshall Space Flight Center, AL 35812, (256) 544-2121

Abstract. This work is supported and managed through the NASA Marshall Space Flight Center - SBIR Program. Studies on cells exposed to microgravity and hypergravity indicate that human cells need gravity to stimulate cell growth. As the gravitational force increases or decreases, the cell function responds in a linear fashion. This poses significant health risks for astronauts in long term space flight. LED-technology developed for NASA plant growth experiments in space shows promise for delivering light deep into tissues of the body to promote wound healing and human tissue growth. This LED-technology is also biologically optimal for photodynamic therapy of cancer.

LED-ENHANCEMENT OF
CELL GROWTH

The application of light therapy with the use of NASA LED's will significantly improve the medical care that is available to astronauts on long-term space missions. NASA LED's stimulate the basic energy processes in the mitochondria (energy compartments) of each cell, particularly when near-infrared light is used to activate the color sensitive chemicals (chromophores, cytochrome systems) inside. Optimal LED wavelengths include 680, 730 and 880 nm. The depth of near-infrared light penetration into human tissue has been measured spectroscopically (Chance, et al 1988). Spectra taken from the wrist flexor muscles in the forearm and muscles in the calf of the leg demonstrate that most of the light photons at wavelengths between 630-800 nm travel 23 cm through the surface tissue and muscle between input and exit at the photon detector. Our laboratory has improved the healing of wounds in laboratory animals by using NASA LED light and hyperbaric oxygen. Furthermore, DNA synthesis in fibroblasts and muscle cells has been quintupled using NASA LED light alone, in a single application combining 680, 730 and 880 nm each at 4 Joules per centimeter squared.

Muscle and bone atrophy are well documented in astronauts, and various minor injuries occurring in space have been reported not to heal until landing on Earth. Long term space flight, with its many inherent risks, also raises the possibility of astronauts being injured performing their required tasks. The fact that the nominal healing process is negatively affected by microgravity requires novel approaches to improve wound healing and tissue growth in space. NASA LED arrays have already flown on Space Shuttle missions for studies of plant growth. The U.S. Food and Drug Administration (FDA) has approved human trials. The use of light therapy with LED's is an approach to help increase the rate of wound healing in the microgravity environment, reducing the risk of treatable injuries becoming mission catastrophes.

Wounds heal less effectively in space than here on Earth. Improved wound healing may have multiple applications which benefit civilian medical care, military situations and long-term space flight. Laser light and hyperbaric oxygen have been widely acclaimed to speed wound healing in ischemic, hypoxic wounds. An excellent review of recent human experience with near-infrared light therapy for wound healing was published by Conlan, et al in 1996. Lasers provide low energy stimulation of tissues which results in increased cellular activity during wound healing (Beauvoit, 1989, 1995; Eggert, 1993; Karu, 1989; Luhart, 1992, 1997; Salansky, 1998; Whelan, 1999; Yu, 1997).

Some of these activities include increased fibroblast proliferation, growth factor synthesis, collagen production and angiogenesis. Lasers, however, have some inherent characteristics which make their use in a clinical setting problematic, including limitations in wavelength capabilities and beam width. The combined wavelengths of light optimal for wound healing cannot be efficiently produced, and the size of wounds which may be treated by lasers is limited. Light-emitting diodes (LED's) offer an effective alternative to lasers. These diodes can be made to produce multiple wavelengths, and can be arranged in large, flat arrays allowing treatment of large wounds. Our experiments suggest potential for using LED light therapy at 680, 730 and 880 nm simultaneously, alone and in combination with hyperbaric oxygen therapy, both alone and in combination, to accelerate the healing process in Space Station missions, where prolonged exposure to microgravity may otherwise retard healing. NASA LED's have proven to stimulate wound healing at near-infrared wavelengths of 680, 730 and 880 nm in laboratory animals, and have been approved by the U.S. Food and Drug Administration (FDA) for human trials. Furthermore, near- infrared LED light has quintupled the growth of fibroblasts and muscle cells in tissue culture. The NASA LED arrays are light enough and mobile enough to have already flown on the Space Shuttle numerous times. LED arrays may prove to be useful for improving wound healing and treating problem wounds, as well as speeding the return of deconditioned personnel to full duty performance. Potential benefits to NASA, military, and civilian populations include treatment of serious bums, crush injuries, non-healing fractures, muscle and bone atrophy, traumatic ischemic wounds, radiation tissue damage, compromised skin grafts, and tissue regeneration.

LED-PHOTODYNAMIC
THERAPY FOR CANCER

Photodynamic therapy (PDT) is a cancer treatment modality that recently has been applied as adjuvant therapy for brain tumors. PDT consists of intravenously injecting a photosensitizer, which preferentially accumulates in tumor cells, into a patient and then activating the photosensitizer with a light source. This results in free radical generation followed by cell death. The development of more effective light sources for PDT of brain tumors has been facilitated by applications of space light-emitting diode array technology; thus permitting deeper tumor penetration of light and use of better photosensitizers. Lutetium Texaphyrin (Lutex) and Benzoporphyrin Derivative (BPD) are new, second generation photosensitizers that can potentially improve PDT for brain tumors. Lutex and BPD have major absorption peaks at 730 nm and 680 nm respectively, which gives them two distinct advantages. First, longer wavelengths of light penetrate brain tissue easily so that larger tumors could be treated; and second, the major absorption peaks mean that more of the drug is activated upon exposure to light. Tumoricidal effects of Lutex and BPD have been studied *in vitro* using canine glioma and human glioblastoma cell cultures. Using light-emitting diodes (LED) with peak emissions of 728 nm and 680 nm as a light source, a greater than 50 percent cell kill was measured in both cell lines by tumor DNA synthesis reduction. The effectiveness of Lutex and BPD against tumor cells in vitro thus established, we have taken the first step toward determining their *in vivo* efficacy by performing experiments to determine the largest doses of both Lutex, or BPD, and light that can be administered to dogs before toxicity is seen, i.e. the maximum tolerated dose (MTD). Using this dose allows us to effect maximum tumor cell destruction during in vivo studies.

For longer wavelengths of light, the improved NASA LED-technology is required. LED's are an effective alternative to lasers for PDT. Laser conversion to near-infrared wavelengths is inherently costly and inefficient, using an argon ion or KTP/YAG laser beam that is converted by a dye module, usually to 630 nm. LED's have been frequently used to emit longer wavelength broad spectrum near-infrared light of 25-30 nm bandwidths. LED lamps traditionally consist of an array of semiconducting LED chips. In recent years, improvements in semiconductor technology have substantially increased the light output of LED chips. A novel type of LED chip is based on the semiconductor Aluminum Gallium Arsenide (AlGaAs). These LED chips have been manufactured to emit light with peak wavelengths of 680 and 730 um, which are optimal wavelengths for the absorption spectrum of the new photosensitizers used for cancer PDT.

Human trials have begun at the Medical College of Wisconsin, Naval Special Warfare Command and NASA- Marshall Space Flight Center.

Photodynamic Therapy with NASA LED Human Subjects

Preclinical studies of LED-photodynamic therapy were reported previously (Whelan, 1993, 1999; Schmidt, 1996, 1999).

The first patient treated with the NASA LED probe in our Photodynamic Therapy Phase TI study, is a 20 year old female who underwent PDT on May 4, 1999 for a brain tumor (anaplastic ependynoma). She had had two previous PDT treatments with **laser** light in another area of the brain. The most recent tumor recurrence formed in a different location of the brain than the previous two sites and is thought to be the result of the laser light not being able to penetrate the tissue deep enough to prevent recurrence. As is evidenced by the graph below (Figure I), LED and photofrin together allow for deeper penetration of tissue, thereby exposing surrounding tissue which may contain stray cancer cells to the LED light.

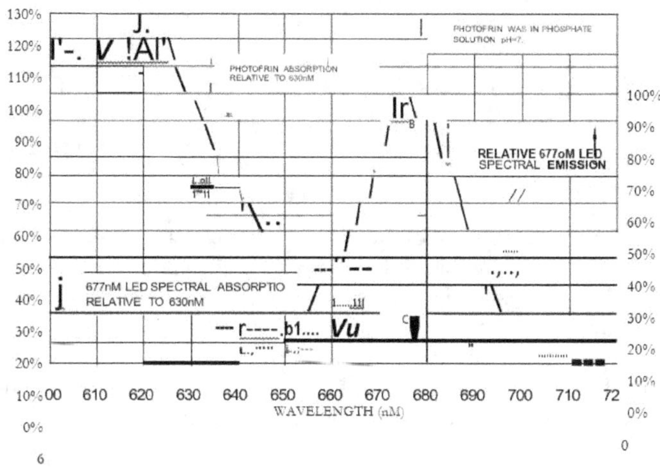

FIGURE 1. Spectral comparison of LED and Photofrin. Photofrin absorption of 677-nm LED relative to 630-nm absorption line. A, Photofrin absorption curve relative to 630 nm. B, spectral emission of the LED. C, integration of the LED spectral emission and the Photofrin absorption.

Post surgically, she experienced some edema as is expected from brain surgery, and was treated successfully, and discharged on May 14, 1999. Follow-up MRI scans do not demonstrate tumor growth. A subsequent 21 year-old male with brain tumor (glioblastoma) was treated August 25, 1999, with LED-photodynamic therapy, he tolerated the procedure well and shows no evidence residual tumor on subsequent neuro imaging.

CP504, Space Technology and Applications International Forum-2000,
edited by M. S. El-Genk

WOUND HEALING WITH NASA LED

Preclinical LED-Wound Healing studies were reported previously (Whelan, 1999).

LED-Diabetic Mice

Type II, Diabetic Mice with excisional skin wounds were treated with LED's at 680, 730, and 880nm, 4J/cm2. LED treatment produced increased healing rates, compared to surgical controls. Refer to table of diabetic mouse data using 4J/cm2 of energy (Figure 2).

A repeated measures analysis was conducted using a General Linear Model with SqrtArea as the dependent variable and Treat as the independent variable. The interaction effect Day *Treat is significant (p-value=0.0095), indicating that there is a significant difference between treatments on some days. This test is of primary interest in this situation, because it shows that the treatments are effective for some part of the treatment period (Figure 2). This analysis was carried out using the SAS statistical software package, published by The SAS Institute, Inc.

The group means are as follows:

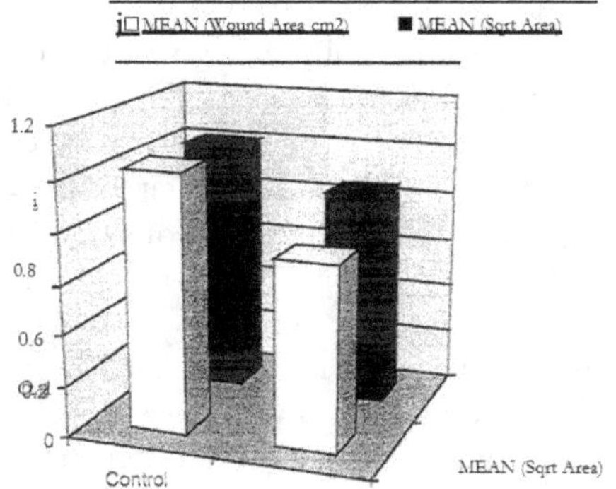

	Control	ELT
ti MEAN /Wound Area cm2)	1.0244	0.7307
■ MEAN fSart Area)	1.0121	0.8548

FIGURE 2. LED-Treatment Wound Area-vs-Control.

Variables

Wound Area   The size of the wound, in cm^2.

SqrtArea   The square root of Wound Area, this is used in the dependent variable in the analysis. This transformation was needed to correct for non-constant error in the General Linear Model. SqrtArea could be interpreted as being proportional to the radius of a circular wound.

ELT   LED External/Light Therapy

LED-Human Subjects

Pt. #1 is a 31 year-old white female insulin dependent diabetic (type 1) with end-stage renal disease status post renal transplant failure and bilateral below knee amputations. Her left amputation site has poor healing compared to the right. She was receiving Hyperbaric Oxygen therapy because of bilateral arterial insufficiency ulcers on her hands. In January of 1999 she had a hangnail on her right third finger and sores developed at the tip. Multiple fissures and sores on both hands further occurred. Sores covered with black eschar developed and her hands are dry with very limited range of motion. She has similar processes on both hands and had similar processes developing on her feet prior to undergoing bilateral below the knee amputations. At that time she complained of cold-induced cyanosis of the fingers and has been developing fissuring of the skin on her hands and some small spots on her fingers. She is a nonsmoker and has been on dialysis for her renal failure. The renal failure and the arterial insufficiency ulcers of her extremities have been felt to be due to vasculitis. She does not use alcohol and has no drug allergies. She had renal transplant for renal failure in 1996 with removal of the transplanted kidney in 1998. She has received Prednisone and Cytoxan for her vasculitis and she also takes Synthroid for hypothyroidism. She has had problems in the past with gastroparesis and had a temporary percutaneous endoscopic gastrostomy tube in place, but has never had a diagnosis of gastroesophageal dysmotility. She has no history of calcinosis and she is anuric because of renal failure. A renal biopsy performed December 5, 1997 of her transplanted kidney showed "focal necrotizing glomerular nephritis, no evidence of acute rejection, no evidence of recurrent diabetic neuropathy". She received 20 treatments of 8 J/cm^2 NASA LED light therapy to all surfaces of both hands. Prior to starting treatment her hands were cold and dusky, lacking sensation. They had many eschar covered ulcerations. After light treatment we noted an improvement in color and hands were warm to the touch. Her complaints of pain and itching indicated a return of sensation.

PT #2 is a 76 year-old white male, borderline diabetic with two open sores on his right medial malleolus. These wounds were traumatic, caused when he was wounded by mortar fire during World War II in the Battle of the Bulge. He has had open sores in that area since that time. These wounds have required two split thickness grafts. One was performed in 1945 and another in 1965. Both grafts have been of questionable success. Mr. Marek has been treated with 52 Hyperbaric Oxygen Treatments to date and has received 19 treatments of 8J/cm^2 of NASA LED therapy to his ankle wound. At the start of NASA LED treatment the area had opened into one large 2cm X 3cm wound draining sanguineous fluid. Since treatment we have seen an increase in tissue granulation from the inside towards the outer edges of the wound. Area has decreased to 1.5cm X 2.8cm and there is a significant decrease in drainage. Transcutaneous Oxygen Measurement (T.C.pOJ readings have shown an improvement in vasculature to the area. (Figure 3)

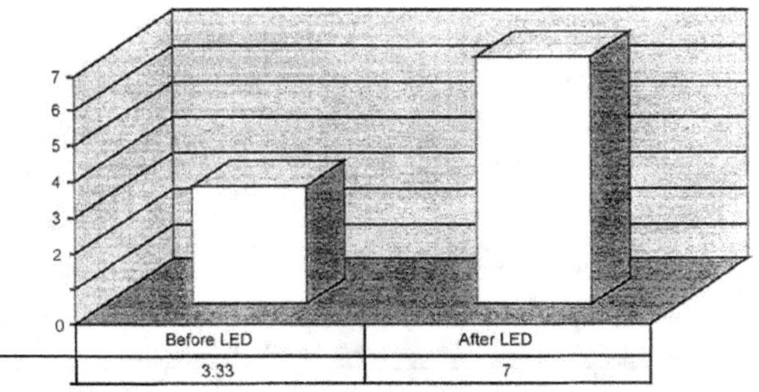

FIGURE 3. Effect of NASA LED Treatment of Ankle Wound Sustained in Combat during WWI I Battle of the Bulge at 8 Joules /cm2 demonstrating improvement in T.C.p0 2 (y-axis).

Further In Vitro LED Cell Growth Studies

In-vitro studies continue with the 3T3 Fibroblasts, and L6 Rat Skeletal Muscle cell line. Stimulation with LED's clearly shows proliferation of both cell lines with the DNA synthesis assay. The first graph below shows the 3T3 Fibroblasts with stimulation of 4 J/cm², 8 J/cm² and 12 J/cm² of energy and proliferation of cells within 3 hours after exposure to LED (Figure 4). The second graph below depicts growth of the L6 Skeletal Muscle over a period of 48 hours after exposure to 4 J/cm² of energy (Figure 5). These data demonstrate *immediate* benefit of LED exposure in-vitro, as in the 3T3 Fibroblasts, but also *over a period of time,* over 48 hours with the L6 Muscle Cells.

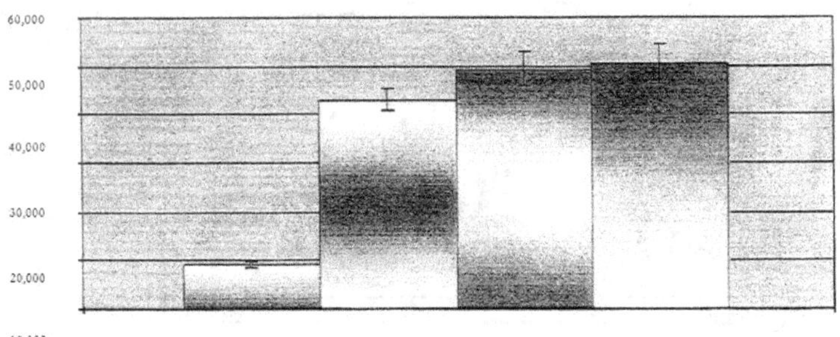

FIGURE 4. 3T3 Fibroblast DNA Synthesis 3 Hour Incubation - LED dose-response 4, 8 & 12 J/cm2.

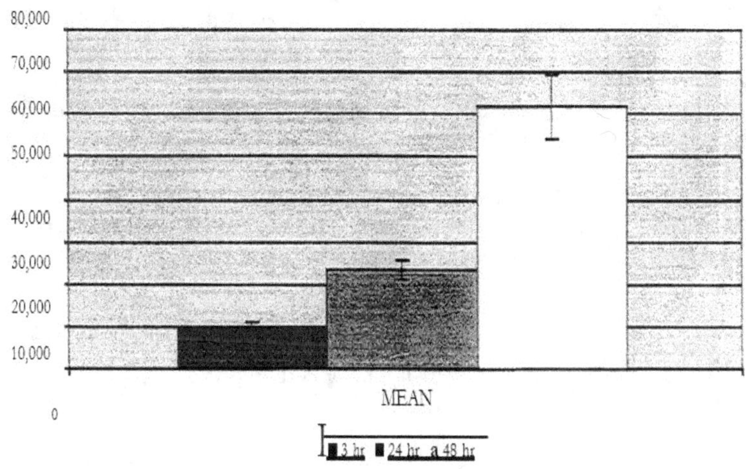

FIGURE 5. L6 Rat Skeletal Muscle - LED-treated at 680, 730 & 880 nm with 4 J/cm2 each.

ACKNOWLEDGMENTS

We wish to thank Karen Zeqiri for assistance in manuscript preparation. The LED arrays were provided by Quantum Devices, Inc., Barneveld, WI. We also gratefully acknowledge the Department of Defense, Air Force Material Command, Armstrong Laboratories, Davis Hyperbaric Laboratory, Brooks Air Force Base, TX for providing the hyperbaric chamber used in this research. The hyperbaric oxygen treatments of our human subjects were performed by Estelle Woodard, C.R.T., and C.H.T. This work was supported by the National Aeronautics and Space Administration, Marshall Space Flight Center SBIR grants: NAS8-99015 and NAS8-97277, Children's Hospital Foundation, the MACC Fund and Quantum Devices, Inc.

REFERENCES

Beauvoit B., Evans S.M., Jenkins T.W., Miller E.E., Chance B., "Contribution of the Mitochondrial Compartment to the Optical Properties of the Rat Liver: A Theoretical and Practical Approach," *Analytical Biochemistry* **226,** 167-174 (1995).

Beauvoit B., Kitai T., Chance B., "Correlation between the Light Scattering and the Mitochondrial Content of Normal Tissues and Transplantable Rodent Tumors," *Biophysical Journal* 67, 2501-25 IO (1994).

Chance, B., Nioka, S., Kent, J., McCully, K., Fountain, M., Greenfield, R., Holtom, G., "Ti me-Resolved Spectroscopy of Ilemoglobin and Myoglobin in Resting and Ischemic Muscle," *Analytical Biochemistry* **174,** 698-707 (1988).

Conlan, M.J., Rapley, J.W., Cobb, C.M., "Biostimulati on of wound healing by low-energy laser irradiation," *J Clin. Period ont.*

23, 492-496 (19 96).

Eggert H.R., Blazek V., "Optical Properties of Normal Human Brain Tissues In The Spectral Range of 400 to 2500 nm,"

Advances in Experimental Medicine & Biology **333,** 47-55 (1993).

Kam T., "Photochemical Effects Upon the Cornea, Skin and Other Tissues (Photobiology Of Low-Power Laser Effects," *Hlth Physics* **56,** 69 I-704 (1989).

Lubart R., Friedman H., Sinyakov M., Cohen N., Breitbart H., "Changes in Calcium Transport in Mammalian Sperm Mitochondria and Plasma Membranes Caused by 780 nm Irradiation," *Lasers in Surg & Med* 21,493-499 (I 997).

Lubart R., Wollman Y., Friedman H., Rochkind S., Laulicht L., " Effects of visible and near-infrared lasers on cell cultures,"

Journal of Photochemistry & Photobiology **12(3),** 305-3 IO (1992).

Salansky N., "Low energy photon therapy for wound healing." Internal Med Instructor, Canadian Defense Ministry, Personal Communication. (1998).

Schmidt M.H., Bajic D.M., Reichert K.W. II, Martin T.S., Meyer G.A., Whelan H.T., "Light-emitting diode s as a light source for intra-operative photodynamic therapy." *Neurosurgery* **38(3)**, 552-556 (1996).

Schmidt M.H., Reichert K.W. II, Ozker **K.**, Meyer G.A., Donohoe D.L., Bajic D.M., Whelan N.T., Whelan H.T., " Preclinical Evaluation ofBenzoporphyrin Derivative Combined with a Light-Emitting Diode Array for Photodynamic Therapy of Brain Tumors." *Pediatric Neurosurgery* **30,** 225-231 (1999).

Whelan H.T., Schmidt M.H., Segura A.O., McAuliffe T.L., Bajic D.M., Murray K.J., Moulder J.E., Strother D.R., Thomas J.P., Meyer G.A., "The role of photodynamic therapy in posterior fossa brain tumors: A pre-clinical study in a canine glioma model." *Journal of Neurosurgery* **79(4),** 562-8 (1993).

Whelan H.T., Houle J.M., Donohoe D.L., Bajic D.M., Schmidt M.H., Reichert K.W., Wcycnberg G.T., Larson D.L., Meyer G.A., Caviness J.A., "Medical Applications of Space Light-Emitting Diode Technology Space Station and Beyond." *Space Tech. & App. Int'! Forum* **458,** 3-15 (1999).

Yu W., Nairn J.O., Lanzafame R.J., "The Effect of Laser Irradiation on the Release Of bFGF from 3T3 Fib roblasts."

Photochemistry & Photobiology **59,** 167-70 (1994).

Project Rebuild Resources

Menopause
https://www.mdanderson.org/publications/cancerwise/7-things-to-know-about-menopause-and-breast-cancer.h00-159306990.html

Estrogen
https://theconversation.com/what-women-with-breast-cancer-should-know-about-estrogens-59787

Phytoestrogens
https://www.medicalnewstoday.com/articles/320630#benefits

Black cohosh
https://ww5.komen.org/BreastCancer/Black-Cohosh.html
https://pubmed.ncbi.nlm.nih.gov/23439657/

Red clover
http://pennstatehershey.adam.com/content

Soy Isoflavones
https://www.cancer.org/latest-news/soy-and-cancer-risk-our-experts-advice.html

Dong Quai
https://www.mskcc.org/cancer-care/integrative-medicine/herbs/dong-quai

Ginseng
https://www.mskcc.org/cancer-care/integrative-medicine/herbs/ginseng-american

Drugs
https://www.drugs.com/
https://www.rxlist.com
https://www.pdr.net/

Selective Estrogen Receptor Modulators (SERM)
https://www.breastcancer.org/treatment/hormonal/serms
https://www.drugs.com/sfx/tamoxifen-side-effects.html
https://www.drugs.com/sfx/toremifene-side-effects.html
https://www.drugs.com/sfx/fulvestrant-side-effects.html

Aromatase Inhibitors (AI)
https://www.breastcancer.org/treatment/hormonal/aromatase_inhibitors
https://www.urmc.rochester.edu/encyclopedia/content.aspx
https://www.drugs.com/sfx/letrozole-side-effects.html
https://www.drugs.com/sfx/exemestane-side-effects.html
https://www.drugs.com/sfx/anastrozole-side-effects.html

Breast Cancer Recurrence Calculators
https://www.tuftsmedicalcenter.org/ibtr/
https://www.mdanderson.org/for-physicians/clinical-tools-resources/clinical-calculators.html
http://www.lifemath.net/cancer/breastcancer/condsurv/index.php

Osteopenia/Osteoporosis:
https://www.nof.org/patients/diagnosis-information/bone-density-examtesting/#content
https://www.spineuniverse.com/conditions/osteoporosis/osteopenia-osteoporosis-there-difference
https://www.iofbonehealth.org/what-is-osteoporosis
https://www.mayoclinic.org/walking-for-muscle-and-bone-health/art-20457588
https://www.ncbi.nlm.nih.gov/pmc/articles/PMC4784773/
https://www.healthline.com/nutrition/15-calcium-rich-foods
https://www.healthline.com/nutrition/build-healthy-bones
https://pubmed.ncbi.nlm.nih.gov/20035439/
https://www.getroman.com/health-guide/vitamin-c-and-bone-health/
https://americanbonehealth.org/nutrition/vitamins-for-bone-health

Bone friendly recipes
iofbonehealth.org/recipes

Bonjour JP. (2011). Protein intake and bone health.
ncbi.nlm.nih.gov/pubmed/22139564

Food and your bones — osteoporosis nutrition guidelines.
nof.org/patients/treatment/nutrition/

Lanou A, et al. (2009). Building bone vitality: A revolutionary diet
plan to prevent bone loss and reverse osteoporosis. New York, NY:
McGraw-Hill Professional.

Nutrition:
iofbonehealth.org/nutrition
https://www.healthline.com/health/managing-osteoporosis/7-day-
osteoporosis-diet-plan#key-nutrients

Osteoporosis nutrition therapy:
sci.washington.edu/info/forums/reports/ADA_OsteoporosisNutrit
ionTherapy.pdf

Osteoporosis prevention eating plan [Fact sheet]. (2012)
intermountainhealthcare.org/ext/Dcmnt?ncid=520489229

Sahni S, et al. (2015). Dietary approaches for bone health: Lessons
from the Framingham

Osteoporosis Study.
ncbi.nlm.nih.gov/pmc/articles/PMC4928581/

Calcium:
https://www.healthline.com/nutrition/15-calcium-rich-foods

Magnesium:
https://www.healthline.com/nutrition/build-healthy-
bones#section9
https://www.medicalnewstoday.com/articles/323349#likelihood-
of-an-overdose

Zinc & Copper:
https://www.spineuniverse.com/conditions/osteoporosis/osteopor
osis-trace-elements-zinccopper

Vitamin D:
https://www.nof.org/patients/treatment/calciumvitamin-d/

Vitamin C:
https://www.spineuniverse.com/conditions/osteoporosis/osteoporosis-vitamin-c-keeping-healthy
https://www.algaecal.com/algaecal-ingredients/vitamin-c/

Vitamin A:
https://americanbonehealth.org/nutrition/vitamins-for-bone-health

Vitamin K:
lpi.oregonstate.edu/mic/vitamins/vitamin-K
https://www.mdanderson.org/cancerwise/7-things-to-know-about-menopause-and-breast-cancer.h00-159306990.html
https://www.healthline.com/nutrition/build-healthy-bones#section5
https://familydoctor.org/condition/osteopenia
https://www.healthline.com/health/osteopenia#can-osteopenia-be-reversed?
https://www.nof.org/patients/patient-support/faq/
https://www.spineuniverse.com/conditions/osteoporosis/osteopenia-osteoporosis-there-difference
Vitamin B12:
https://americanbonehealth.org/nutrition/vitamins-for-bone-health

Collagen:
https://www.healthline.com/nutrition/build-healthy-bones#section7

Omega-3 fatty acids:
https://www.algaecal.com/expert-insights/why-omega-3-fatty-acids-are-crucial-for-healthy-bones/

Protein:
https://nutrition.org/meetings/continuing-education/protein-bone-health/
https://journals.lww.com/nutritiontodayonline/fulltext/2019/05000/optimizing_dietary_protein_for_lifelong_bone.5.aspx

Medication for Bone Health:
https://www.drugs.com/zometa.html
https://www.breastcancer.org/treatment/druglist/zometa
https://www.drugs.com/sfx/zometa-side-effects.html

Osteonecrosis:
https://www.breastcancer.org/treatment/side_effects/osteonecrosis
https://www.medscape.com/viewarticle/883371_2
https://rarediseases.org/rare-diseases/osteonecrosis/
https://rothmanortho.com/specialties/conditions/avascular-necrosis-osteonecrosis
https://emedicine.medscape.com/article/1447355-overview

Fatigue:
https://www.sleepfoundation.org/articles/melatonin-and-sleep

Hot Flashes:
Black cohosh
https://ods.od.nih.gov/factsheets/BlackCohosh-HealthProfessional/
https://www.mskcc.org/cancer-care/integrative-medicine/herbs/black-cohosh

Red clover
https://www.nccih.nih.gov/health/red-clover
https://www.mskcc.org/cancer-care/integrative-medicine/herbs/red-clover

Dong Quai
https://www.healthline.com/health/dong-quai-ancient-mystery
https://www.mskcc.org/cancer-care/integrative-medicine/herbs/dong-quai

Siberian Ginseng
https://www.mountsinai.org/health-library/herb/siberian-ginseng
https://www.mskcc.org/cancer-care/integrative-medicine/herbs/siberian-ginseng

Kava
https://www.mskcc.org/cancer-care/integrative-medicine/herbs/kava

Constipation:
https://www.healthline.com/health/constipation-medication#otc-medications
https://www.healthline.com/health/constipation-medication#prescription-medications

Skin & Hair:
https://www.aad.org/public/everyday-care/skin-care-secrets/anti-aging/skin-care-during-menopause
https://crescobar.neora.com/

Weight Gain:
https://www.breastcancer.org/tips/nutrition/after_treat/lose_weight

Natural Aromatase Inhibitors:
https://www.healthline.com/health/low-testosterone/anti-estrogen-diet-men
https://www.healthline.com/health/estrogen-in-men#whats-typical
https://www.ncbi.nlm.nih.gov/pmc/articles/PMC3074486/
https://www.bensnaturalhealth.com/blog/sexual-health/natural-aromatase-inhibitors/
https://www.healthline.com/health/estrogen-blockers-for-men#natural-estrogen-blockers
https://www.healthline.com/nutrition/saw-palmetto-benefits
https://www.nccih.nih.gov/health/saw-palmetto
https://www.ncbi.nlm.nih.gov/pmc/articles/PMC5846366/

CBD/Medical Marijuana:
https://www.breastcancer.org/treatment/comp_med/types/medical-marijuana

Light Therapy:
https://thequantumacademies.com/

Food lifestyles
Mediterranean
https://www.everydayhealth.com/mediterranean-diet/guide/
https://www.heart.org/en/healthy-living/healthy-eating/eat-smart/nutrition-basics/mediterranean-diet
https://www.medicalnewstoday.com/articles/324221
https://www.healthline.com/nutrition/mediterranean-diet-meal-plan

Whole Food, Plant Based
https://nutritionstudies.org/whole-food-plant-based-diet-guide/
https://www.forksoverknives.com/how-tos/plant-based-primer-beginners-guide-starting-plant-based-diet/
https://www.healthline.com/nutrition/plant-based-diet-guide#overview

Vegan/Vegetarian
https://www.medicalnewstoday.com/articles/325478
https://vegsoc.org/info-hub/definition/
https://www.vegansociety.com/go-vegan/definition-veganism
https://www.healthline.com/nutrition/vegan-vs-vegetarian#TOC_TITLE_HDR_6

Keto
https://www.dietdoctor.com/
https://www.healthline.com/nutrition/ketogenic-diet-101
https://www.healthline.com/nutrition/ketogenic-diet-foods

Juicing
https://timesofindia.indiatimes.com/life-style/health-fitness/weight-loss/5-juices-that-will-help-you-lose-weight-in-no-time/articleshow/62069949.cms
https://www.healthline.com/nutrition/can-juicing-help-you-lose-weight
https://juicerecipes.com/juicing/weight-loss-recipes/
https://www.modernhoney.com/healthy-juice-cleanse-recipes/

Carnivore
https://www.healthline.com/nutrition/carnivore-diet
https://carnivoremd.com/the-carnivore-diet-start-here/

Paleo
https://paleoleap.com/paleo-101/
https://thepaleodiet.com/what-to-eat-on-the-paleo-diet-paul-vandyken
https://www.healthline.com/nutrition/paleo-diet-meal-plan-and-menu

https://www.everydayhealth.com/diet-nutrition/the-paleo-diet.aspx

Appetite Suppressants
Gymnema Sylvestre
https://www.verywellhealth.com/gymnema-sylvestre-4692940
https://www.drugs.com/npc/gymnema.html
https://www.healthline.com/nutrition/gymnema-sylvestre-benefits

Konjac Root
https://www.ncbi.nlm.nih.gov/pmc/articles/PMC3892933/
https://www.dietspotlight.com/glucomannan-review/
https://www.healthline.com/nutrition/glucomannan#dosage
https://www.medicalnewstoday.com/articles/319979#summary
https://www.healthline.com/health/konjac#konjac-risks-andprecautions

Over the Counter
https://www.dmagazine.com/sponsored/2020/06/best-appetite-suppressant/
https://fitterliving.com/best-appetite-suppressants/

Lipoic Acid
https://www.ncbi.nlm.nih.gov/pmc/articles/PMC5523816/
https://primewomen.com/health/nutrition/lipoic-acid-and-weight-loss/
https://www.nutraingredients-usa.com/Article/2020/08/13/Lipoic-acid-supplements-may-aid-weight-control-for-obese-people
https://www.sciencedaily.com/releases/2020/08/200812094902.htm

Alli
https://www.verywellfit.com/alli-weight-loss-pills-3495278
https://www.healthline.com/nutrition/alli-diet-pills-review

Leanbean
https://leanbeanofficial.com/

Zotrim
https://zotrim.com/
https://www.ncbi.nlm.nih.gov/pmc/articles/PMC4344557/

https://patents.google.com/patent/EP1037644A1/en
https://pubmed.ncbi.nlm.nih.gov/15930480/
https://pubmed.ncbi.nlm.nih.gov/23207186/

https://pubmed.ncbi.nlm.nih.gov/11424516/
https://www.ingentaconnect.com/content/mcb/070/2007/000001
09/00000006/art00001
https://pubmed.ncbi.nlm.nih.gov/15657469/
https://www.researchgate.net/publication/265379734_Yerba_Mate
_Illex_Paraguariensis_ingestion_augments_fat_oxidation_and_energ
y_expenditure_during_exercise_at_various_submaximal_intensities

Garcinia Cambogia
https://www.ncbi.nlm.nih.gov/pmc/articles/PMC5143754/
https://www.healthline.com/nutrition/garcinia-cambogia-weight-
loss

Prescription weight loss pills
Phentermine Hydrochloride
https://www.healthline.com/nutrition/phentermine-weight-loss
https://www.drugs.com/phentermine.html
https://pubchem.ncbi.nlm.nih.gov/compound/Phentermine-
hydrochloride

Qsymia
https://www.drugs.com/qsymia.html

Orlistat
https://www.drugs.com/orlistat.html

Exercise
https://primewomen.com/health/fitness/moderate-exercise/
https://primewomen.com/health/fitness/muscle-matters/
https://www.sciencedirect.com/science/article/abs/pii/S00917435
16300160
https://www.everydayhealth.com/fitness-pictures/amazing-
benefits-of-exercise.aspx

Workout Plan
Adapted from the U.S. Army, the U.S. Navy, and many amazing
Veterans.

Cancer Trauma
https://www.breastcancer.org/research-news/many-women-have-
ptsd-symptoms-after-dx
https://www.psychologytoday.com/us/blog/all-is-
well/201711/pstd-can-hit-women-breast-cancer-years-after-
diagnosis

www.ingramcontent.com/pod-product-compliance
Lightning Source LLC
Chambersburg PA
CBHW061343250726
48657CB00004B/1310